TAKE CHARGE *of Your* CANCER

TAKE CHARGE
of *Your*
CANCER

The Seven Proven Steps to Healing &
Recovery from Cancer

NORMAN PLOTKIN

NEW YORK

LONDON • NASHVILLE • MELBOURNE • VANCOUVER

TAKE CHARGE *of Your* CANCER
The Seven Proven Steps to Healing and Recovery from Cancer

Published in New York, New York, by Morgan James Publishing in partnership with Difference Press. Morgan James is a trademark of Morgan James, LLC.
www. MorganJamesPublishing.com

The Morgan James Speakers Group can bring authors to your live event. For more information or to book an event visit The Morgan James Speakers Group at www.TheMorganJamesSpeakersGroup.com.

ISBN 9781683509813 paperback
ISBN 9781683509820 eBook
Library of Congress Control Number: 2018934768

Cover & Interior Design by:
Christopher Kirk
www.GFSstudio.com

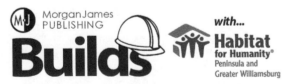

In an effort to support local communities, raise awareness and funds, Morgan James Publishing donates a percentage of all book sales for the life of each book to Habitat for Humanity Peninsula and Greater Williamsburg.

Get involved today! Visit
www.MorganJamesBuilds.com

ADVANCE PRAISE

"Great book. Although I do not have cancer, I found the book very intuitive and enlightening. I think the 7 principles can be used in many facets in life, not just for cancer patients. Very well-written. Very introspective. Great job. Great read."

Linda M Tincher, DDS

"Norman eloquently puts in writing the simple keys to defeating cancer, something that I also discovered along my post-diagnosis and recovery journey. Those of us who have survived our diagnosis, treatment, and recovery have discovered the simple truths and walked a similar path, which Norman lays out in *Taking Charge of Your Cancer*.

Not everybody discovers these truths. Norman takes his research, personal experience, and love for mankind and presents to you, dear reader, what he has discovered – what many survivors have discovered. In short, I consider this book to be a manual... a roadmap... a guiding hand to living with and defeating cancer.

So I ask: Do you want to defeat this diagnosis? Do you want to live another 20, 40, or 60 years? That is not a preposterous question! If your answer is yes, you MUST read this book."

Stephen W. Hogarth, M.Ed., *Pensacola, FL*
GySgt, USMC (Retired)
Colon Cancer Survivor (December, 2004)

"I am impressed! Norm doesn't pull any punches challenging us to take charge of our health. I suggest you skip this book if you get a scary diagnosis and want to just blame others, feel sorry for yourself, or be angry. Read it if you want solid information to maximize your odds for survival and good health. Norm gets right to the point with a blend of memoir, research and actionable steps in 90 easy-to-read pages. His story is about fighting cancer, but he shows us the tools for prevention and healing of every type of disease."

Dorothy Rothrock, *Sacramento, CA*

"Norm Plotkin's empowering and practical program will change your life. *Take Charge of Your Cancer* is a must-read if you are struggling with cancer, seeking to heal, or simply just seeking an effective strategy to live a more meaningful life."

Jean Keese, *McCall, ID*
Clinical Ayurvedic Practitioner, Wellness Advocate & Coach

"Norman is a living example of mind over matter, aka courage over cancer. This is a profoundly powerful must-read about the triumph of the human spirit."

Jann Taber, *Sacramento, CA*

"This book offers an excellent narrative of the author's battle with cancer and how he has chosen to take charge and you can, too.

Whether or not you or a loved one have been diagnosed with cancer *Take Charge of your Cancer* summarizes the 7 steps of healing and recovery most of us can benefit from. The book will provide insight into personal struggles, our health care system, diet, exercise and spirituality. A great addition to your library that offers life enhancing changes."

Explore, Listen and Heal.
Tina Mitchell, Kimberly, ID

To David: You have inspired me in so many ways over the many years, and this book is just the latest example. I am in eternal gratitude for the 22 years that you were my earthly brother and for the immeasurable gift you gave me in your passing. You were the first of my unwrapped gifts, and I look forward with relish to the day when we meet again.

FOREWORD

Rarely does a book so sweet land in a reader's lap. This book is a letter from your guardian angel, written vicariously through an author awakened by his own cancer story and sent to you. This book is here to guide you, warn you, empower you, and help you protect yourself on your healing path, a path seemingly with threats around every corner.

And the threats are many. The author has been dealing with threats for decades. Formerly a lobbyist for Fortune 500 companies, Norman Plotkin had wined and dined with the politically powerful until God claimed him and sent him cancer to wake up. The Creator put him on his knees and made him look the beast in the eye... and the truth he learned has been delivered to you here in this book.

If you are not okay with being passive in your own healthcare, if you are not okay with seeing yourself reduced to a helpless victim, if you are not okay with being misinformed and led like a sheep for slaughter, this book is for you. If you don't buy into an idea that cancer just happens to you and you personally can do nothing about it besides obeying instructions and handing over your body into the hands of a massive industry that profits from your *helplessness*, this book is for you. If you don't want to volunteer to become just another experiment when someone is merely *practicing* medicine – an art that defies mastery and is completely subjective – this book is for you. If you are too intelligent to surrender your ability to ask questions and question everything that's spoon-fed to you as truth, this book is for you. If you know that nothing can kill human spirit like a dire expectation and if you are even remotely open to exploring the power of the mind when it comes to creating disease as well as healing it, this book is for you. If you are conscious enough to take responsibility for your life and own it, ha! This book is for you!

Written with love, eloquence, and extensive research, *Take Charge of Your Cancer* empowers you to do just that: become the captain of your healing and recovery, become the boss of your treatment. After all, it is your own body, your own health, and your own life that are at stake. And, just like when it comes to money, no one will take care of your health better than you, when you are in charge.

You will learn about the way your mind has been involved in the creation of your cancer and about the way it can also participate in the dismantling of it. Yes. You are that powerful.

In my work with cancer clients, I have witnessed a lot of healing miracles and rapid recovery taking place. They would apply a strict fasting protocol and raw vegan diet. And, there was always a time when they would reach a plateau, and it was apparent something stood in the way of their progress and was not allowing them to heal. They would just settle for *feel better, good enough*, and return to old ways of living and eating. Cancer would return as well. Like a boomerang.

Watching how desperately their body wanted to heal, and how swiftly it was making progress, regaining its strength when relieved by detox and exposed to healthy, plant-based nutrition, I wondered what was missing. Was there something that could help to engage their mind, as it was obviously the only obstacle and stumbling block that remained, often full of excuses? I wondered if there was a way to repair their psychology, amend their emotional health, and release all the irrelevant, heavy-duty stories they were telling themselves over and over like a broken record.

After the years, it became clear to me that all the cancer patients I'd ever met and talked with had had a traumatic experience that occurred in their lives before they were diagnosed. Something terrible happened – one event was enough, but sometimes they were cumulative. A betrayal of a loved one, a financial crisis and overwhelming debt, the loss of a child or dream job, a disappointment or rejection, a relationship filled with guilt, blame, and shame. That something unleashed a chain of events that, like an avalanche of bad luck, became unbearable to the subconscious.

I used to watch their souls trapped in their stories, and ask, *What are you trying to get out of by creating cancer?*

An inquisitive investigator and a talented hypnotherapist, Norman Plotkin has combined all of the pieces, building on the excellent and detailed work of many leaders in the field of medicine, psychology, spirituality, nutrition, and healing, and has written a plan of action that sprang from the pages of his own experience. This book is the missing piece that I had struggled to help my clients with in the past.

You can now stand on the shoulders of those who have gone before, learn, and avoid so many of the common mistakes people make because they just don't know and confine themselves to the tumor model of cancer treatment that typically just involves surgery and chemical and radiological therapies.

We've been waiting for it!

Evita Ramparte
Solana Beach, CA
September, 2017

Evita Ramparte is a Polish investigative journalist who explores the truth about human health, wellness, performance, and sexual vitality. A former TV news reporter, bestselling author, Cosmopolitan *and* Newsweek *contributor, and health and wellness expert, Ramparte was also featured in the movie* Hungry for Change *and the* Food Heals *Podcast.*

TABLE OF CONTENTS

INTRODUCTION

*"There is one consolation in being sick; and that is
the possibility that you may recover to a better state
than you were ever in before."*

Henry David Thoreau

What if I told you that you could reframe cancer to be a challenge rather than a threat? Life whispers to us, and if we do not hear it, or, worse, if we ignore it, life will yell at us. When this yell takes the shape of illness, it is a message to change. The challenge and message of cancer is a siren call, an opportunity to undergo personal growth. In this personal growth lies the prospect for true and lasting healing.

I'm not alone in seeing my cancer as an opportunity for personal transformation. Many cancer patients use the experience as a turning point to expand contemplation through techniques like meditation; to radically change their diet; to deepen their spiritual connection; to follow their intuition and establish rapport with their subconscious; to release suppressed emotions; to take control of their health; and to embrace a reason to live instead of a fear of dying. These are the people who survive and thrive.

My mother had a plaque that hung in the hallway of our house when I was a kid that read: *The journey of a thousand miles begins with a single step*. The saying seemed so simple at the time. In retrospect, a single step is a deliberate move, a conscious act. Too often, our journey begins the way I was taught to swim at two years old: thrown in the water and told to find the side, reach and pull, kick, kick, kick.

I swallowed a lot of water. And I barfed. But I learned to swim.

And so, our journeys begin, often less with a deliberate step and more with a plunge, reaching and pulling, kick, kick, kicking.

And you swallow water. And you barf. And sometimes you are so busy keeping your head above water that you miss the wonder, the beauty of life in what truly is a paradise if you only have eyes to see it.

And sometimes you miss the gifts that life has given to you because they are unwrapped, disguised before your very eyes but in plain sight if you have the right perspective.

There is a Taoist saying that the journey is the reward. Insofar as the journey itself is rewarding, it can be made more so when you embrace a perspective of gratitude that will allow you to see gifts in all of your experiences, even those that on their face might seem awful, even tragic.

But in order to get to the place where you can have this kind of perspective, you need to know yourself. While this may seem obvious, think for a moment about the fact that in modern society, we have drastically reduced the use of our senses for survival, and so they are being diminished. We turn instead to external sources like the Internet, which is perpetually at our fingertips on our increasingly powerful personal devices, and we rely on government and institutions for health and safety. When sick, we turn ourselves over to a medical community that usually removes patients from the planning process while the experts decide what is wrong with our bodies and decide what to do in order to fix them.

There is a school of thought, however, that is characterized by the belief that the body has an innate, intuitive knowledge regarding what it needs in order to heal. Those who subscribe to this belief system believe that the body can also let you know why you got sick in the first place. And while there are powerful lessons to be learned from your own body if you listen, you must be careful regarding your thoughts simply *because* you are listening.

You are reading this book because you have cancer, or you know someone with cancer, or you do not want to become a cancer statistic and would rather make changes in your life and behavior that will lead to a healthy and vibrant immune system, capable of doing its amazing work repelling the external threats posed by the toxicity of our environment and surroundings. If you have cancer, you are undoubtedly overwhelmed by the very notion of the diagnosis, as well as the world of scientific, evidence-based medicine and decisions such as the surgical, chemical, and radiological therapies that make up the tumor model of Western medicine. And while it can be very reassuring to have highly trained, competent, and talented medical professionals doing their professional, medical best to get you to a positive outcome and a restoration to quality of life, they don't go home with you at night when the questions really cross your mind and the doubt and fear can creep in.

Adding to this disjointed, episodic care is the fact that medical professionals, by training, remain at arm's length. If they didn't, they couldn't cope with the enormity of all of their patients' hopes and fears. And because so much of medicine today is scientific and seemingly beyond the layperson's ability to understand, the medical community tends to be a bit paternalistic and reluctant to involve patients in their own treatment plans. There is a tendency to just go along with the program, to do as you're told and be optimistic.

Because of these underlying conditions, you are likely and rightly feeling like, *I don't want to be a helpless victim, so I'm looking for direction in order to play an active role in my own healing and recovery.* Intuitively, you know that your active engagement will increase your chances of survival and recovery. But engagement isn't part of the tumor model of medical therapy for cancer, a model that includes tests, scans, surgery, radiation, and chemotherapy. Nevertheless, your intuitive desire to take an active role in your treatment is the first step in establishing the foundation for your *healing and recovery and a return to your normal life.*

I know this because I am a cancer survivor. In 2011, I was diagnosed with papillary carcinoma and underwent a radical thyroidectomy and nodal neck dissection (five lymph nodes removed), followed by two rounds of radiation therapy. I rode the roller coaster of fear, anxiety, depression, and the gamut of other emotions that accompany a cancer diagnosis. Along the way, I had teachers and guides appear, and I learned to listen to my intuition. The single biggest thing I learned was that no one had more skin in the game than me, and my survival depended on me taking control of my healthcare plan and making changes in my life. In short, I needed to *take charge of my cancer*.

In the following pages, I will share my story and what I learned from it. Further, because the experience was such a life-changing event, I will share what I have found in my research during my recovery, research that has yielded a framework for action on your part that has the power to lead you into healing and recovery.

CHAPTER 1
MY WAKE-UP CALL

"Action cures fear, inaction creates terror."
Douglas Horton

I was raised on a ranch, and from an early age adopted a pretty solid work ethic. I worked hard and played hard. I did not go directly to college after high school, opting instead for the Marine Corps. When I got out, I went to work on a drilling rig and worked at various other oil field jobs. When the price of oil dropped and the fields were shuttered, I went to work at a rock plant making little rocks out of big rocks, kind of like Fred Flintstone, operating various pieces of heavy equipment. About the time I had mastered every process at the quarry, there was a change of ownership, and I used that as an excuse to move on. I then went to work for a cable television company in the small community where I had grown up in the southern Sierra Nevada Mountains of California. I had moved from in-house with the cable company to subcontracting and was toiling along when my younger brother was killed in a car accident.

David, a pre-med student at the University of California, San Diego, was just about to turn 22, and then, in the blink of an eye, he was gone. I struggled tremendously with his death. Here was the person with whom I had spent almost every day, every holiday, and every event of my life. Sure, we fought, and as he got bigger than me he challenged me as all *little* brothers do. But it soon became apparent that if we continued down that route, someone was going to get seriously hurt, so we settled into a fantastic adult brother relationship. And now he was gone.

I struggled emotionally, eventually closing my contracting business and moving back in with my mom. I tried to find meaning in this tragedy, but there was only a vacuum. And then one day it occurred to me that even if I could not find meaning in my brother's death, I could use this tragedy to better myself in his memory and in his honor.

I started college and finished in less than four years, despite long hours spent participating in student government and speech and debate. At the end of my junior year, I was hired as a clerk in the state legislature. After finishing school, I went on to work for a total of 10 years in the legislature – first as clerk, then legislative assistant, and finally as committee consultant to the Assembly Health and Insurance Committees.

I left the legislature to work as a lobbyist for the California Medical Association (CMA). As a lobbyist for the CMA, I represented physician interests before the legislature by analyzing legislation and influencing the respective measures through meetings with legislators and staff, correspondence, and committee testimony in ways that were consistent with the perspective of physicians. I learned a lot about the modern practice of medicine from the physicians themselves, as well as the development of public policy in the health field. Little did I know that this experience with medical policy and physicians and the world of modern health care delivery would be valuable preparation for navigating the fight of my life.

After several years with the CMA, I struck out on my own, establishing my own contract-lobbying firm. I represented clients in the energy, automotive, and petroleum industries. I loved developing strategy for clients who faced threats from prospective legislation, and I loved the public policy development process. Because of my experience as a clerk, I knew the rules like few others, and because I had run campaigns along the way, I knew the politics. I really enjoyed creating client campaigns to influence legislation.

Before I knew it, I had been at it for 10 years. But years eight and nine were in the aftermath of the economic downturn, and client budgets were reduced, which meant that there was less money for things like lobbyists. About the same time, politics changed. Politics has always been a rough and tumble sport, but in my opinion, the political climate just seemed to get mean and nasty. Another factor that perhaps influenced this shift was that term limits, passed in 1990, finally swept all of the pre-term limits legislators out of office. Regardless of your perspective on term limits, an indisputable result was that there were a lot of new people, and many old relationships were now no longer relevant.

Representing clients before the legislature and state agencies was a stressful career to begin with, but these changes in the landscape made things more difficult and more stressful. There was a lot at stake. And the legislative process, at least in California, which is really a nation-state with an economy that ranks seventh in the world, is deadline driven with most bills being heard in long hearings at the deadline and the end of session consists of weeks of around the clock activity. After more than 20 years, I was used to it. But with the added stress of managing the business in the softened economic climate and having to work harder to build new relationships, I began having a hard time keeping up. It was initially most noticeable with my ice hockey team.

And then something terrible happened, which, in a book about fighting cancer, is saying a lot. As you will read later in Chapter 5, high-stress events can have an emotional impact that lodges in our subconscious and lays the groundwork for subsequent illness. The following event threatened my very livelihood and, as a result, adversely affected my subconscious. This subconscious impact very likely set off a chain of physical events that ultimately impacted my immune system's ability to function properly.

Every two-year session, lobbyists must take an ethics training class. I had been through them numerous times as a lobbyist, and before that, I had been through them as a legislative staffer. But this particular year, I waited until the last offering and then had a conflict when a client measure for which I had to appear and give testimony came up at a regional Air Resources Board meeting in Los Angeles (the ethics training was in Sacramento). There was no provision for make-up or remote attendance. I went with the client appearance and missed the training. I proactively attempted to make it up after, but was denied. Turns out the Secretary of State was a former state senator who I had tangled with in her committee during testimony on a very controversial bill, and she wasn't about to do me any favors. Within weeks, I was notified that my lobbyist registration was revoked, and a letter went around to all legislators and staff that a number of lobbyists were suspended for failure to attend ethics training. I wasn't the only one, but this was of little consolation.

Eventually I appealed, was allowed to remotely attend the training, and was reinstated as a lobbyist. But the highly visible, embarrassing experience in an industry where perception is reality, coupled with the timing, took a severe toll on me. I experienced extreme fatigue and gave up hockey all together. I stopped riding my mountain bike. I did continue playing golf, but my game sucked because I couldn't get out of my own head. I saw the doctor, and he took me through a lot of tests. When statins failed to control my high cholesterol and I began experiencing brittle fingernails and thinning hair, he sent me for an ultrasound of my thyroid.

The ultrasound showed that I had a nodule on my thyroid. The doctor said very little by way of background, other than that we would continue to monitor it. I did a little cursory research and found information on goiter, but the Internet had far less information available then than it does now. I just knew I didn't want a big growth bulging out of my neck! They measured it every three months for *two* years. All this time I didn't feel well, I didn't sleep well, and I was on an emotional roller coaster.

During this time, my wife's brother died of a heart attack at 52 years old. Her whole family was angry at his wife for not trying to do more for him during the attack, and they were blaming her. It was a very difficult time. As far as my condition, the doctor finally told me that we needed to wait until the nodule got to three centimeters. He tried putting me on thyroid hormone therapy, but it just made me feel weird, so I told him I didn't want to take it. I felt increasingly out of sorts, with fatigue, night sweats, and irritability. I found it very difficult to console my wife over her family difficulties as I struggled with my own physical and emotional challenges, and the relationship became strained.

Then my wife's brother-in-law was diagnosed with pancreatic cancer. I had golfed with him in February, and he had complained of unexplained back pain. When I saw him on St. Patrick's Day, he was jaundiced and looked like he had lost 40 pounds. It was just three months from his diagnosis until he passed away. My wife was overcome with grief, and her doctor prescribed pills for her anxiety and depression. Her father had died when she was seven and now, the two men who had acted as surrogates for her growing up were both dead. In addition to the pills, she was drinking more than usual.

My primary care physician had given me a number of scenarios up to this point about what might be going on with me, and most of them sounded like routine stuff. Just to be sure, the doctor ordered a scan. So, I presented myself to the radiology department, where I was given a gown that ties in the back and seated outside the advanced radiology rooms along a wall with 12 other scantily clad people, mostly women, who all looked a little pale and didn't even attempt small talk.

The clinic had overbooked the CT scanner worse than United Airlines, and I spent almost two hours waiting for my scan. The woman next to me had gotten up three or four times to check to see if her turn was close. Finally, she announced to no one in particular that she had to pick up her son from school because she had no one who could do it for her, so she left after having waited for two hours and had to be scanned another day. I felt really bad for her, but like everyone else in the hallway, I said nothing.

Two weeks after the scan, the doctor called and suggested that I make an appointment with another doctor for another procedure. The scan was inconclusive, the doctor said, but there appeared to be some atypical cells, so they wanted to poke the nodule and have a closer look at the cells. A pathologist poked me with a long needle, known as fine needle aspiration, and another couple weeks went by; I was starting to wonder what might be really going on. At the same time, I was feeling less energetic than my usual self, and promised myself that I was going to get to the gym and work out. And work seemed more stressful than ever. This was particularly difficult because I was not sleeping well, waking many times per night with night sweats.

Finally, my doctor called again and said that they weren't sure what to make of the atypical cells. They wanted me to go to another specialist, an endocrinologist. At this next appointment, the specialist reiterated that the cells were atypical and said that he wanted me to see a surgeon. Finally, I thought, *someone is going to do something*. The surgeon will just cut out the "atypical" cells and we can get back to normal, get life back on track.

The surgeon was a kind man from India, and he was accompanied by a young resident. He said that I had papillary carcinoma of the thyroid and that he wanted to remove my thyroid completely. I asked if complete removal was necessary, and he said yes, that was what was indicated because there was a very strong likelihood that once diseased, the organ would continue to produce malignancy. I asked when he was thinking about doing the surgery, and the resident said we should do it right away. I understood the sense of urgency she was trying to convey with her nonverbal emphasis, so I scheduled the surgery for two weeks out and drove home in a fog.

I felt like I had been punched in the gut. Numerous scenarios were discussed up to this point, but the word *cancer* had never been uttered. The surgeon wanted to schedule the surgery next week. Four doctors into this experience, and this was the first anyone had said anything about *cancer*. Why wouldn't they say the word?

The surgeon gave me an old, poorly photocopied list of resources, including the Cancer Society, the Thyroid Cancer

Society, support groups, web links, etc. A million thoughts raced through my mind. My inner marine wanted to fight! But how? I didn't even know where to start. Even with all of my experience with the healthcare system and the fact that I knew hundreds of doctors, I felt anything but in control of my care. Instead, I felt more like a shuttlecock in a nightmarish game of badminton.

I researched the surgeon and found that he went to medical school in India. I thought about seeking another surgeon, someone trained in the United States. I thought, like most people, that doing something meant trying to choose the best doctors. But then I had a meeting with my intuition, which told me everything I needed to know: that this physician was highly skilled and possessed a kindness that obviated any concern over where he went to school.

As a kid on the ranch, I rode bulls in junior and high school rodeos. I participated in extreme sports like hang gliding and "jump, turn, or die" snow skiing. I climbed Mount Whitney. I was a marine. I had never known fear. Suddenly, I got a taste of raw fear. The thing about raw fear is that it isn't a single taste; it is accompanied by the mother of all esophageal reflux, which keeps bringing it up for another taste so that it is constantly with you.

The next week I was involved in a lobbying coalition that defeated a bill sponsored by a major car company that would have hurt my automotive aftermarket clients. It was a nice victory to experience right before the legislature broke for summer recess and I went under the knife, as they say. My close friends wondered how I was remaining so calm. I just said there wasn't much more you can do. I didn't tell them that the feeling I had when told I had cancer, that feeling of being punched in the gut, never went away, instead lingering as a constant reminder and accompanied by that fear reflux.

The surgery – a thyroidectomy and a lymph node dissection – went well, or so I was told. My wife was by my side for the overnight stay and tended to me thoughtfully. But through the haze of morphine, I was a little perturbed at the young nurse who, upon seeing my wife help me use the bedpan, asked if she was my daughter. This gave me the impression that I wasn't looking so good, since my wife was only four years younger than me. Nevertheless, in fairly short order, I was back home playing with my young kids and trying to regain strength.

Without a thyroid, my metabolism was off, which had all kinds of implications and would for several weeks, as they wanted me completely devoid of thyroid hormone for my first scan. Nonetheless, I had client comments due on the Cap and Trade measure, and a week after my surgery I wrote 24 pages of comments to the Air Resources Board. I was really proud of myself for mustering the fortitude to draft these detailed comments, and the effort had the effect of reassuring me that I still had my mental faculties as well as my fortitude and work ethic. It also didn't hurt that my clients thought I was a machine for delivering so soon after my surgery.

Two weeks after the surgery, I tried to attend a client board meeting and had a martini at the reception the first night, which was a huge mistake. I couldn't metabolize the alcohol, spent a miserable sleepless night, and drove home the next morning. For all of the bolstering effects of getting substantive, detailed comments written and submitted for my clients so soon after the surgery, this experience of a sleepless, restless night where I felt like a stranger in my own body took me in the opposite direction and left me wondering what my post-cancer future would look like.

Several weeks later, I was given a radioactive iodine pill and then scanned. Since the only organ in the body that takes up iodine is the thyroid, the scan showed to what extent any residual tissue remained. The pill would cause the residual tissue to decay, or ablate, as it was operated on by the retained radioactive iodine. The experience was a bit unnerving, as the physician entered a small room with the pill in a lead container and then exited very quickly after telling me to open the container and take the pill only after he cleared the room.

Because I was weeks out from having thyroid hormone, I felt like I was a 78 record being played at 45 (for those too young to know what that means, I was in slow motion). I had to be isolated for three days while radioactive. Neighbors and family members cooked for us and watched our kids; everyone was very helpful and loving.

Time passed. My healthcare providers assured us of an excellent prognosis and told us that papillary carcinoma is well understood, well differentiated, and generally responds well to treatment therapies. What my wife heard was, *if you have to have cancer, it's the best kind.* She was ready to get back to normal as if nothing had happened, and in fact, began to act as though it never happened. She didn't want to talk about it, and she certainly didn't want to mention anything about it in front of the kids. What I heard was, *if my cancer didn't respond well, distal metastasis went to bones and lungs.* I wanted recognition that I wasn't out of the woods yet.

The problem was that I didn't feel well. I was severely hypothyroid without the organ, I wasn't taking replacement hormones, and I was feeling pretty awful from the radiation. Then the doctor started me on thyroid replacement and didn't explain that they start you out with what they call suppression therapy – in other words, on a high dose in order to trick the body into not thinking itself thyroid deficient and, therefore, regenerating thyroid tissue.

I went from severely hypothyroid in slow motion to severely hyperthyroid with my metabolism at high speed: I was sweating, I wasn't sleeping, I had heart palpitations, and I was irritable. I would walk the block from my office to the capitol in the late summer heat and be soaked in sweat, with dark circles under my eyes. When trying to give testimony, as I had done hundreds of times, my mouth got dry and my heart raced in my chest.

One of the many things that medical providers don't tell you, or at least not in my experience, is that the disease doesn't just affect you. You never know how others in your life and particularly your family members will react to the cancer experience generally, and to your day-to-day struggles with the disease and its treatment on you specifically. Support groups are suggested and so is counseling, but these can feel like complicated layers on top of everything else you are dealing with. At the time, I simply didn't understand how important these tools were for creating understanding. It is so very important to address the family dynamic. In retrospect, my focus on myself, while understandable, meant I may have failed to understand the impact my illness was having on my wife and see that she could have benefitted from counseling.

The agitation that I was experiencing as a result of hyperthyroidism left me feeling frustrated and detached from my body, and led my wife to withdraw further and to pretend nothing had happened. As described, she was already on at least two different pills and drinking regularly, and soon I began to join her. It felt like the only thing we could manage to accomplish together, even though alcohol was terrible for me.

At six months, my doctors took me off the hormone in anticipation of my next scan. Predictably, in retrospect, I whipsawed from hyper- to hypothyroid, and became a wreck of a different color. The scan confirmed what I knew and had been trying to convince my wife of: the cancer had come back, and I was going to need another round of radiation.

Just before the scan, my wife asked if I was going to manage my son's baseball team again that year. I had done so for several years, but I just wasn't up to it this time, as I was feeling weak and fatigued. I told her to stay involved and be the team mom. Unfortunately for me, she took my advice a little too much to heart and had an affair with the coach who replaced me. I might have been hypothyroid, but I wasn't blind or stupid. And if I thought I was gut punched when told of the cancer, this blow doubled me over, followed closely by an uppercut. I went into my second round of radiation feeling more alone than ever before in my life. The three days of isolation I spent in a motel room, required because the radioactive iodine that I ingested made me and my bodily fluids radioactive and therefore a danger to anyone who might come into contact with me, were some of the most desperate of my life. I'll never forget my kids waving to me through the motel window.

I tried to haul my wife into counseling, but by then she'd checked out of the marriage. Men in her life died when they got sick, and it was just a matter of time, she thought, before I'd do the same. She was just a little early replacing me. The term *adding insult to injury* just does not do justice to how this marital betrayal made me feel. I vacillated between righteous indignation and a level of woundedness that flattened me, and left me wondering how I was going to take on both cancer and infidelity at the same time. I obsessed over the looming loss of all of my material things: the big house, the cars, the toys, the lifestyle. Mixed in with the fear was anger over how someone who took vows of *in sickness and in health* could not just desert, but betray me in my hour of need. It would take me five years to forgive her.

Yes, I thought briefly about taking my own life – it felt like I was losing just about everything – but it passed. I quickly came to the conclusion that it didn't matter how tough things got for me, I wasn't going to do that to my kids. I then found an old friend who had gotten out of politics and opened a yoga studio. She was the first of many teachers who appeared to help me take charge of my own healing. I can safely say that Jean saved my life! She took me through therapeutic yoga for cancer. On days when my mind was swirling between images of my cheating wife and the internal ravages of radiation treatment, she sat me down and guided me through meditation with sound therapy of bowls or oms. She taught me Ayurveda practices such as eating for my pitta dosha, abhyanga (oil massage), and how to regain strength through Pilates, because by that time, I was an emaciated, atrophied mess.

Jean gave me reading recommendations like the works of the Dalai Lama, Carolyn Myss, and Wayne Dyer. And then, as Dr. Dyer has famously said, as I changed the way I looked at things, the things I looked at changed. I moved to Los Angeles and went back to school. Along the way, I attended a Hay House Conference and saw Myss, Dyer, and so many other amazing, inspirational healers speak. I reconnected with a girl who I'd known since we were 11 and who I'd dated briefly in high school, and began a new relationship.

I looked for meaning in the things that happened to me, just as I had when my brother was killed. I was led to a book called *Man's Search for Meaning* by Viktor Frankl, a psychiatrist and holocaust survivor who founded what he calls *Logotherapy*, in which he suggests that there are three avenues to meaning in life: 1) creating a work or doing a deed; 2) experiencing an event or encountering someone (love); and, most importantly (according to Frankl), 3) turning our predicaments into achievements by rising above hopelessness and growing beyond ourselves.

It was within this context that I was satisfied that things happen for a reason (didn't hear life's whisper) and that meaning is found if we can rise above our predicament and grow beyond our former self. When I finished school, I became a certified hypnotherapist. Today, I'm also certified in many other specialties, including hypnotherapy for cancer clients and helping people unlock the power of their subconscious mind for healing and recovery.

I have expanded my hypnotherapy practice to coach cancer clients on the powerful tools that I have learned the hard way and that I have found to have been substantiated by research. Tools that all survivors utilize to recover and heal. I found my way to these practices and have incorporated them into my life, but only because I stumbled upon an old friend who pointed me in the right direction. Even with this nudge, it has been a long, disjointed, and painful journey. Sometimes I find myself wishing I could have found an easier path, found a guide or a resource that could have saved me some of the agony along the way. And then I realize that it happened exactly how it was supposed to happen, and that my growth is demonstrated by my service to others.

This service to others includes doing the research for this book and developing a program to teach the seven tools for healing and recovery. My cancer experience was a lesson and a gift that I was given, in order to help people like you make the changes that will lead to healing and avoid some of the mistakes and pitfalls that people can make when they are overwhelmed by a disease that doesn't care that you also have to go on living *and* making a living *and* being a family member, on top of fighting for your life.

Ultimately, I discovered the meaning of life is to find your gift even when it is unwrapped, and the purpose of life is to give the gift to others. This book is my effort at giving my gift to you, so that you can learn from what I have learned and apply it in your life in order to take charge of your cancer and, as a result, make the behavior and lifestyle changes that will lead to healing and recovery.

CHAPTER 2
COMMON THREADS OF SURVIVAL

"I found it shocking that the vast majority of academic articles did not mention what the patients thought might have led to their remissions. I read article after article by doctors who carefully listed all the biochemical changes the Radical Remission survivors experienced, but none of the authors reported directly asking the survivors why they thought they had healed."

Kelly A. Turner, Ph.D.

A year before he died of pancreatic cancer, my brother-in-law, Mark, told me he'd read an article that suggested that within eight years, everyone diagnosed with cancer would survive because medical treatments would have advanced so significantly and early detection would have continued to increase. He was encouraged that survival rates had already increased, and thought that in the foreseeable future, cancer would not be eliminated, but would be declassified from the scourge that it has been in the modern era.

The problem for Mark was that his malignancy was not detected until stage four, and after distal metastasis to surrounding organs. Even that might not have been a conclusive factor had he engaged himself in his own healthcare plan in the three months from the time he was diagnosed until the time that the medical professionals removed life support after complete organ failure. But that isn't part of the tumor model of cancer treatment in Western medicine, and Mark and his family knew of no alternatives. Instead, he and his family were in high-stress response, made no lifestyle or diet changes, and turned Mark over to the medical community in complete surrender, becoming virtually demoralized by no-hope prognoses, as they traveled around seeking expert opinions from renowned specialists in the fervent wish that someone who would tell them something different from what they'd heard. The result was the *expectation* of a dire prognosis and imminent demise, and that is exactly what unfolded. I would give anything to turn back the clock and share with Mark what I have learned. His death hit me hard because I felt so helpless for him. I hated the way he was treated by a one-dimensional medical approach.

Expectation plays a huge role in healing. Mark was given the *expectation* of no hope, and so this became his reality. This could also have been what was going on with my doctors who, perhaps tacitly addressing expectation, wouldn't tell me I had cancer until I scheduled the surgery for its removal and they needed informed consent. I would have liked to have had a frank conversation with a physician earlier in the process about the possibility. In either case, expectation is an important element. So, let's take a look at what is behind expectation in the healing process.

The placebo effect is well known and acknowledged by Western medicine. You know, fake treatments such as sugar pills, saline injections, and similar techniques. These techniques are routinely used in clinical trials as a control against which drugs, treatments, or surgeries are measured in order to determine if they are truly effective. In a landmark 1955 study by Dr. Henry Beecher featured in the *Journal of the American Medical Association* and titled *The Powerful Placebo*, about a third of people who were given inert ingredients like salt water or sugar, for example, were not only cured in their minds, but also showed measurable physiological recovery.

In modern, evidence-based medicine, any drug, treatment, or surgery must do better than the placebo in trials in order to be deemed effective. So, the power of the placebo effect is not only acknowledged by evidenced-based medicine, it is used as a baseline determinant for what is considered an effective therapy. But it poses a practical problem for a doctor in modern practice, who, as Deepak Chopra has noted, considers the placebo effect a nuisance because their medical training has preconditioned them to consider *real* medicine as drugs and surgery, and their medical ethics preclude prescribing *fake* drugs.

But people like Dr. Chopra and others argue that the placebo effect *is real* medicine because it triggers the body's healing mechanism, and it does so, free from side effects. Every thought, decision, and action influences a chemical feedback loop within the body. For these reasons, it is critical to be aware of your self-talk and your thoughts because, as the placebo effect makes very clear, *expectation* plays an incredibly important role in your healing and recovery.

Conversely, just as you can positively influence your healing, you damage your body's natural state of health or worsen your disease condition with negative thoughts. The fact that this input comes from the brain means that thoughts, moods, and expectations, incorporeal and detached as they may seem, get translated into chemical messages just as surely as chemical therapies like drugs. You *must* be deliberate in your thinking, because it is your responsibility and in your self-interest to send positive messages to your cells as opposed to negative ones.

Expectancy plays a tremendous role in your day-to-day health, but it is especially powerful when you are sick and/or in a diseased state. It has been scientifically proven that focusing your attention on illness will make you sick. Ask any medical student if, after accumulating substantial knowledge about what can go wrong with the body and the endless ways in which the physical body can break down, they didn't at least once begin to experience physical symptoms. A 1966 study in the *Journal of Medical Education* titled *Medical Students' Disease: Hypochondriasis in Medical Education* found that 79 percent of students reported developing symptoms.

This phenomenon has been referred to as the *nocebo* effect. Where the placebo effect reinforces the power of nurturing, hope, positive thinking, and expectation, the nocebo effect points to the power of negative thinking and how it can cause one to experience physical symptoms. In either case, we see the power of expectation, state of mind, and the foundation for the mind-body connection.

The Big C

A quick search of WebMD tells us that cancer, also called malignancy, is an abnormal growth of cells. There are more than 100 types of cancer, including breast cancer, skin cancer, lung cancer, colon cancer, prostate cancer, and lymphoma. Symptoms vary depending on the type. Cancer treatment may include chemotherapy, radiation, and/or surgery.

Forty-six years after President Nixon declared war on cancer, a recent study published online in the journal *JAMA Oncology* reported that cases rose 33 percent worldwide in the past 10 years. In 2015, there were 17.5 million diagnoses and 8.7 million cancer deaths worldwide. The *Global Burden of Disease Cancer Collaboration* study found, among other things, that the lifetime risk of developing cancer was one in three for men and one in four for women.

According to the article's author researcher Dr. Christina Fitzmaurice from the University of Washington in Seattle, prostate cancer was the most common type of cancer in men (1.6 million cases), and tracheal, bronchus, and lung cancer were the leading causes of cancer death in men. Breast cancer was the most common cancer for women (2.4 million cases), and was also the leading cause of cancer death in women. The most common cancers in children were leukemia, other neoplasms, non-Hodgkin's lymphoma, and brain and nervous system cancers. Cancer is the second leading cause of death worldwide.

In January 2017, Rebecca Siegel, strategic director for Surveillance and Health Services Research at the American Cancer Society, released the latest cancer incidence and mortality estimates, which indicate that in 2017, over 1.3 million Americans will be diagnosed with cancer and about 600,000 US cancer patients will die. Siegel noted that the decline in cancer mortality is primarily the result of large drops in the four major causes of cancer death: lung, colorectal, breast, and prostate, which account for almost half of all cancer deaths.

So, as worldwide cancer cases are increasing, at least the mortality rate in the United States is declining, due in large part to reduced smoking and earlier detection efforts, but it remains nearly a 50-50 proposition. Is it any surprise then that some patients view a diagnosis as a death sentence?

Even the most optimistic, positive-thinking person diagnosed with cancer is fraught with stress and anxiety upon diagnosis. At the same time that they enter a state of shock, in complete stress response, fight or flight, autonomic nervous system overload, they have equal amounts of information overwhelm thanks to the Internet and a medical community that counsels removal of the patient from the planning process and relegates them to a subject of the experts' determinations as to what is wrong with their body and how the medical professional is going to *fix* it.

At this point, the newly diagnosed cancer patient and their loved ones, whether they realize it yet, or not, *want to understand how they can play an active role in their treatment and recovery.* But as noted, engagement isn't part of the tumor model of medical therapy for cancer, which fairly universally includes tests, scans, surgery, radiation, and chemotherapy. Yet, we have an intuitive desire to take an active role in our treatment, and this is the first step in establishing engagement and expectation, which are exceedingly important because they set the stage for the Pygmalion effect, or Rosenthal effect, which is the phenomenon whereby higher expectations lead to an increase in performance.

There are nascent efforts at developing integrative medicine departments (also called complementary or alternative medicine departments) within hospitals and health institutions that provide patient participation-oriented modalities and therapies, but little education and outreach is done to engage patients in the active participation of these offerings that include energy healing, hypnotherapy, yoga, meditation, and acupuncture, to name a few, and for which there is promising research that validates the efficacy of such treatments.

As research is done and empirical studies substantiate the mind-body connection, leaders in the medical community are taking notice. Lissa Rankin, M.D., has written an insightful book called *Mind Over Medicine, Scientific Proof That You Can Heal Yourself,* in which she comes from a classically trained physician's perspective to reveal what she calls the shocking truth about your health beliefs. She goes on to detail how to manage your thoughts in support of that mind-body approach, and finishes with how to write your own *prescription* for healing. Dr. Rankin also discusses the concept of spontaneous remission and points to the work of Kelly A. Turner, Ph. D., and her seminal research that gave rise to her book, *Radical Remission, Surviving Cancer Against All Odds*. In *Radical Remission*, Turner, a researcher and psychotherapist who specializes in integrative oncology, shares the amazing research she has undertaken studying thousands of cases of radical remission, which she refers to as people who have experienced a complete reversal of serious and/or terminal cancer diagnoses.

These books really resonated with me because for the first time in my experience, I was finding that people were writing about alternative ways to see and approach cancer. Although these books weren't written until years after my diagnosis, the conclusions correlated with my own experience and underscored that the same things that I did to improve my condition have been demonstrated to work for others. The only difference is that I found them the hard way.

That timing can be ironical is not lost on me. I wish I had found Turner's book for Mark, or when I was first engaged in my own cancer journey. Unfortunately, my cancer journey began before its publication, and before the Internet began to recognize and popularize movements like integrative medicine and functional medicine, modalities that evidence-based medicine had previously referred to as complementary and alternative medicine (CAM) and cautioned against by the conventional medical community.

Nevertheless, just as the article Mark had referenced suggested, while much progress is being made in the fight against cancer by conventional means such as early detection, as in my experience, we are also seeing that if we can be powerful participants in our own care, we can create the dynamic of positive expectancy and trigger immune response through mind-body communication – another powerful lesson for me. Turner defines a radical remission as any cancer remission that is statistically unexpected and facilitated by not using any conventional medicine; or having tried conventional medicine with no effect, switched to alternative treatment that did lead to remission; or a combination of conventional and alternative treatments that lead to outliving a statistically dire prognosis (< 25 percent chance of survival beyond five years).

What Turner, as well as works like Dr. Andrew Weil's *Spontaneous Healing,* Dr. Rankin's *Mind Over Medicine,* and Deepak Chopra's *Quantum Healing* tell us is that there are statistically significant actions we can pursue that every person who was studied because of their remission results undertook. What is remarkable is that we are talking about thousands of unrelated cases that were not coordinated, and yet these actions were consistently taken across the board. Some of these actions are obvious and some are not, but all are somewhat intuitive if you have the right frame of mind. Miraculously, I found my way to these actions, but not because any of my doctors recommended them.

Turner's study is important on its face because these are remarkable stories, but it takes on an even greater significance within the context of mind-body healing and the validity of integrative measures, and will help you transcend your opinion of illness generally and cancer specifically. Suddenly, you have documentation that treatments once considered "alternative" actually work, either alone or in conjunction with the tumor model of evidenced-based medicine. The numbers are too significant to relegate the phenomena to the junk heap of the unexplained spontaneous event. Nor do the evidence-based medicine terms for spontaneous remission: psychosomatic and placebo effect adequately account for the efficacy of mind-body integrative measures. Now, studies are emerging quantifying mind-body immune response. Psychobiology and psychoneuroimmunology give us a chemical explanation for what was previously unexplained. We begin to understand the limbic-hypothalamic system as the mind-body information transducer and modulator of the autonomic, endocrine, and immune systems.

While this is not a text book or medical manual, nor am I a physician, a brief quote from *The Psychobiology of Mind-Body Healing* by Ernest Lawrence Rossi should lay to rest any questions about the physiological explanation and provide evidence that our mind can affect our body chemistry:

> *"If you push any endocrinologist hard enough he or she will admit that … under "mental stress" the limbic-hypothalamic system in the brain converts the neural messages of mind into the neurohormonal "messenger molecules" of the body. These, in turn, can direct the endocrine system to create*

> *steroid hormones that can reach into the nucleus of different cells of the body to modulate the expression of genes. These genes then direct the cells to produce the various molecules that will regulate metabolism, growth, activity level, sexuality, and the immune response in sickness and health."*

In other words, your brain chemistry can be altered by your mental state to convert hormones in your body chemistry that can change your genes and affect your body's subconscious response from your metabolism and immune system.

Despite this scientific explanation, evidence-based medicine remains reluctant to fully embrace mind-body methodology. Perhaps it is because medical schools approach the human body basically as a machine. The machine is then segmented into its working parts – i.e., cells, tissue, and organs. When the body breaks down through illness, something material is at fault. Although modern medicine goes into elaborate scientific detail, it is essentially interested in two basic principles, which are materialism and reductionism. A physical explanation for every phenomenon is required in materialism; and all solutions and answers to complex problems are derived from breaking the problem down into its component parts. Where evidence-based medicine gets tripped up is in the demarcation of the brain, which is material and quantifiable, and the mind, which is esoteric or metaphysical, the realm of philosophers, not scientists. This is the foundational question of consciousness and the plane on which we can influence our outcomes.

In his book *Quantum Healing*, Deepak Chopra, M.D., proposed an innovative framework for describing and understanding this division between brain and mind. Borrowing from the scientific cousin world of physics, Chopra described the sub-atomic, invisible domain of the *quantum field* in physics known as a jump to a higher level of function, and suggested that just such an invisible quantum field was the domain of the mind-body connection. Nearly 30 years after its first publication, *Quantum Healing* is far less controversial than when it was written, but retains critics from the world of evidence-based medicine. Imagine scientists trying to get their head around the notion that the brain was creating the mind and the mind was creating the brain, simultaneously!

Dr. Chopra explored the question of why healing as expressed by the body's mending of a broken bone is any different than the healing expressed by a spontaneous remission of cancer, and answered by suggesting that conventional medicine holds that the broken bone seems to heal by itself, without the intervention of your mind, yet a spontaneous remission of cancer is widely believed to depend on some miraculous will to live or some rare capacity, with the implication that there is *normal* healing and *abnormal* healing, which he rejects. I reject this notion and you should reject this notion, too. Instead, he believes that both occur on a conscious level. To get to the quantum state of healing, Dr. Chopra argues that you must move past the material level of the body and push to the junction of mind and matter, where consciousness begins to have an effect. Having healed from both a broken arm and from cancer, I cannot consciously differentiate between the two experiences because there is no *normal* healing and *abnormal* healing. Dr. Chopra was being nice. If you think about it for a moment, the notion of abnormal healing is preposterous.

All of this says that you are capable of making a conscious decision to heal, which has been scientifically shown to influence your body's chemistry, which in turn influences gene expression and molecular communication, and which in turn influences your immune system. Studies have shown that there are thousands of cases where people from all over the world and from all walks of life have included in their conscious decision to heal a number of conscious actions. So, it seems pretty logical and important that these actions should be pretty universally undertaken by someone diagnosed with cancer who wants to do everything they can to survive the challenge. Amazingly, even though I didn't know I was doing it at the time, I did just that, and as a result, am here to write about it. You can, too!

Before we expand on the behavioral changes proven to effectively round out the tool chest for the cancer patient who wants to take charge of their healthcare plan and be an active participant in their healing process, let's consider for a moment a 2008 MD Anderson Cancer Center finding that only 5-10 percent of all cancer cases can be attributed to genetic defects – meaning that 90-95 percent are rooted in lifestyle and the environment. The specifically cited factors included cigarettes (yes, people still smoke even with all we know about the health effects of smoking), diet (specifically fried foods, red meat, and sugar), alcohol, sun exposure, environmental pollutants, infections, stress, obesity, inflammation, and physical inactivity.

With such an overwhelming influence on health from lifestyle, it should come as no surprise that making lifestyle and behavioral changes immediately is the first act of taking control of your health care plan and involving yourself in your healing process, thus, *taking charge of your cancer*. Unfortunately, I didn't understand this right away, and it wasn't until I had the cancer return and a second round of radiation was necessary that I finally came to understand that my role included some behavioral and lifestyle changes. In *Radical Remission*, Dr. Turner noted nine common actions recoverees undertook that they believed led to their outcome. Doctor Rankin, in *Mind Over Medicine*, detailed six that overlapped the nine. And then there is *Cancer: 50 Essential Things To Do*, by Greg Anderson. I have taken the nine from *Radical Remission*, consolidated a couple, and come up with the seven things that it just so happens that I did during my cancer journey.

It is from the groundbreaking works referenced above that these steps have emerged, steps that all of the studied survivors incorporated into their healing regimes and which the following pages will detail.

Some, including myself, have stumbled upon these steps, but at significant cost in physical and emotional terms that you can avoid by your early adoption. These healing factors are each a component of a systematic approach to engaging in your own healing process, creating an expectation of healing, and transforming your perception of the disease from threat to challenge. These steps are:

Meditation

It may seem rather obvious that the two most prominent conditions that accompany a cancer diagnosis are stress and anxiety, but what do you do about stress and anxiety? If you are like most people these days, you get a prescription, but that is not the kind of healthcare plan that is going to yield any significant results and, in fact, may exacerbate your condition. Instead, healing begins in the mind, at the exact moment that we establish ourselves as in charge of our illness. The first step in the healing process, once decided and in charge, is to get control of your mind-talk, or self-talk.

All of your experiences, memories, and stored information stimulate the main activity of your mind and translate into self-talk. While you collect negative experiences, you also create capabilities for attention, concentration, mindfulness, and meditation, which you, like everyone else, rarely use because it requires effort. You express your self-talk through thoughts, images, sensations, and feelings, creating attitudes and behaviors that impact your daily life. Unhealthy self-talk leads to powerlessness as well as her step-sisters helplessness, inadequacy, and loneliness, which are experienced as isolation and deprivation. These states are generally marked by self-talk that leads to emotional distress, anxiety, worry, and fear. You need to learn to take control of the predominantly automatic mental chatter that is self-talk; you need to take control by learning to practice mindfulness and learning meditation. Mindfulness and meditation are the first steps toward self-regulation and will allow you to find peace by relaxing your mind and body. Meditation is a powerful tool to gain control of self-talk, which is the foundation for the following processes.

Diet

As the MD Anderson report demonstrated, diet is a huge influence on the development of illness, specifically cancer. But diet has an equally central role in healing. You must see nutrition as medicine and the fuel to recovery. This means healthy eating, understanding food influences on cancer, and committing to permanent dietary changes. Obesity, nutrient-sparse processed foods such as concentrated sugars and refined flour products that contribute to impaired glucose metabolism (which also leads to diabetes), low fiber intake, consumption of red meat, alcohol consumption, and imbalance of omega-3 and omega-6 fats all contribute to excess and ongoing cancer risk. Portion control is another important mindset change.

Spirituality

Spiritual eyes allow us to see value in all of the simple things in our life, even during times of challenge and difficulty. The cancer patient who opens their mind and spirit can transcend the cancer experience and make a connection to personal spiritual growth. And the signs of spiritual growth are unconditional love, gratitude, and forgiveness. There are many paths to the divine, but no path to recovery is without a spiritual component.

Subconscious

The subconscious mind is the route through which your body knows what it needs to heal and recover. Getting into rapport with your subconscious through listening to your intuition and experiencing hypnotherapy will unlock powerful tools that you already possess. With your cancer diagnosis comes a deep, multilevel crisis associated with anxiety. You must confront fear of death at the same time that physical and emotional pain associated with chemotherapy, radiation, and invasive surgical procedures combine to take a severe toll on your immune system. Hypnotherapy can be used to increase the immune response. It can also be instrumental in transforming negative perceptions you may have formed during times of uncertainty that may be blocking efforts to reverse the illness. You want to make sure the powerful, goal-oriented machine that is your subconscious is playing a properly supportive role in your healing journey.

Emotion

Holding on to the unresolved hurt that led you down the illness path must be identified, and let go of. Stress, trauma, fear, regret, anger, and sadness are all negative emotions that, when unresolved, fester and compromise our immune system's ability to fight disease. Your recovery is heavily influenced by your ability to release what no longer serves you.

The other side of the emotional coin is the development of strong, positive emotional practices. When we are happy, our bodies are flush with healthy immune cells – seems obvious, right? The neurotransmitters produced when positive emotions are experienced powerfully boost your immune system.

Taking Charge

As noted, healing begins the moment you decide to take control of your health. Taking responsibility as well as engaging and changing behavior are the keys to sustainable health and recovery. You can have the greatest physicians who will give you unmatched care in a supportive environment, but you see them in a snapshot in time and at the end of the visit, you go home and must contend with your illness in a continuous, real-time loop. As the manager of your own care, self-care is a built-in component, and it is an important one.

Reason to Live

Finally, it is not enough to not want to die; this is a negative perspective with a focus on dying, which leads to fear. You must want to live. Create your expectations and have reasons to live. Amazingly, the six preceding steps will have set the stage for this step because now you will be a happy, mindful, healthy-eating, non-stressed manager of your healthcare and your subconscious mind. The only thing left to do is embrace and return the love of your social support system and nurture your relationships.

CHAPTER 3
EYE OF THE STORM

"The experience of inner peace is my true gauge of all accomplishments."
Wayne Dyer, *Living the Wisdom of the Tao*

What exactly is mindfulness meditation? A *Perspectives on Psychological Science* study described mindfulness meditation as *the nonjudgmental awareness of experiences in the present moment*. Another study notes that the psychological benefits of mindfulness training on emotion regulation are well documented, but the precise mechanisms underlying these effects were unclear. They proposed a link between mindfulness and improved emotion regulation that signifies the role played by executive control. Specifically, and with a trigger warning that a dense, evidence-based scientific explanation follows, they suggested that the present-moment awareness and nonjudgmental acceptance that is cultivated by mindfulness training is crucial *in promoting executive control because it increases sensitivity to affective cues in the experiential field. This refined attunement and openness to subtle changes in affective states fosters executive control because it improves response to incipient affective cues that help signal the need for control. This, in turn, enhances emotion regulation.* In presenting their model, they discussed how new findings in executive control can improve our understanding of how mindfulness increases the capacity for *effective emotion regulation.* (Teper, Segal & Inzlicht 2013)

What?!? The paragraph above characterizes the Western medicine attempt to explain what is going on in meditation, but efforts like this miss the point of meditation altogether. For meditation to be effective, you are going to need to forget about the dorsal anterior cingulate cortex, the executive control network and the capacity for emotion regulation in the experiential field. But then Western progress of knowledge has historically been based on outward observation, not inner.

Meditation has been referred to as a fourth state by the Indian *rishis*, a state that is neither waking, nor sleeping, nor dreaming, and because it is outside normal experience will allow you to cut through all illusion, all projection, and all confusion you have about yourself and about others. But in order to reach this fourth state, your mind must transcend its normal activity. Remember, all of your experiences, memories, and stored information stimulate the normal activity of your mind and translate into your self-talk. The problem is that this mind activity is influenced by perception and amplified by emotions. You are always thinking, and most of the time you are experiencing emotions. But your thoughts don't mean anything; they are not who you are. Thoughts naturally come and go all of the time, but when you attach yourself to your thoughts, you can and likely will, experience suffering.

Meditation is about coming *face-to-face* with your mind. Understand that this will lead you to penetrating insight into the illusions you have created in self-talk through the some-times-distorted process of emotionally amplified perception. Have you ever been like me and worked yourself to inaction when your overactive mind imagined every possible scenario and every possible negative outcome in a game of high speed, mental ping-pong? People usually imagine that meditation is a technique that will train them to throw a psychological switch that will turn off the thinking and self-talk activity and leave the mind blank, calm, peaceful. I did. That is not how it works. Initially, thoughts, self-talk, and mental activity will continue. What changes is how you respond to it. This was an incredibly valuable lesson that I learned.

The end of that penultimate sentence bears repeating: what changes is how you respond to it. In order to arrive at that point where healing begins in your mind, the exact moment that you establish yourself as in charge of your illness, you must get control of your self-talk through the exercise of meditation as a first step in changing how you respond to your illness. The good news is that you have the capabilities for attention, concentration, mindfulness, and meditation. You have deployed attention and concentration in school, at work, and perhaps at play, but you are proba-bly not as familiar with meditation and mindfulness, so they might be initially challenging because they require effort. When I began, I was like Julia Roberts' character in *Eat, Pray,*

Love, frustratingly trying to sit still and quiet my mind with my eyes closed. We all are, and it's ok. The important thing is to stick with it.

The danger for you as someone battling cancer is that unhealthy game of mental self-talk ping-pong can lead to powerlessness marked by self-talk that leads to emotional distress, anxiety, worry, and fear. This is why meditation is such a critical tool to be used as a method to change the predominantly automatic mental chatter that is self-talk.

The effort to learn meditation is so worth it because not only does it help you control your thoughts, images, sensations, and feelings that create your attitudes and behaviors, but also your ability to control these mental features will have a direct and profound impact on your healing and recovery. The irony is that you, like everyone else, rarely give much thought to thinking, it is an automatic process that can go wayward if you aren't deliberate. Have you heard the saying *change your thoughts, change your life*? But when you first try meditation, as you sit and concentrate on your breath, a thought will arise. Before you realize it, you are involved with the thought; you get caught up in it and begin to develop elaborate follow-up thoughts. Before I developed discipline (over years of practice building to my current hour a day meditation practice), I could be ten levels of thought into a distraction, with six degrees of separation from the original thought and where I ended up.

As an example of how it can go, you may have had an innocent thought about breakfast. Immediately, you are off to the races thinking about over-easy or omelet, cage-free eggs (oh they're all cage free in California because of that ballot proposition a couple years ago – that's why they're so expensive), bacon or sausage, wheat or white toast, etc. Two things happened: an innocent initial thought, and then the elaboration. It is the latter that is the distraction. The initial thought is gone in an instant; the elaboration can continue for minutes, hours, days or even *years*. This activity that you generally think of as *thinking* can hold you in a type of bondage, a slave to your lost-in-thought process that transports you forward or backward in time, robs you of your present moment, and keeps you from living in the here and now. Worse, it can leave your mind weakened, confused, dull, and scattered.

This is where most people bail out and determine that meditation and mindfulness are not for them. But you don't have that luxury. And your thoughts are likely far less mundane than what's for breakfast, you are thinking about appointments with specialists, medication, upcoming procedures, and so on – thoughts with a far greater gravity than eggs or oatmeal. What you need to do, and it comes with practice, is learn to drop the thought and return to the present, keeping the mind open, relaxed, and loving. Do not criticize yourself; rather, disengage. With practice, you will make a liberating discovery. You will find it possible to feel the freedom of not being bound by compulsion to endless thought by just letting the thoughts and feelings drop.

From experience, I know that when you are in the throes of illness, you can get caught up in whirling, recurrent thought patterns that endlessly repeat. This is known in psychological terms as obsession. Obsessive thinking can be exhausting, and when taken to logical extremes, it can be terrifying. Your diagnosis has an enormous emotional content, and the thought of its details and implications will tend to flood into the mind frequently and without invitation. You get sucked into the powerful emotions surrounding these thoughts, and this can create a confused fog. The practice of meditation and the act of letting go will lead you back to the object of meditation, the present moment, and to the discovery that freedom and peace are available to you.

Let's have a look then at what the first step in your seven-step process of taking charge of your health, meditation, looks like. It is safe to say that the biggest impediment to getting into meditation is distraction. Distraction comes in three parts: following the past, getting spun up in the present, and engaging in the unending planning or thinking about the future. When you start meditating, you will find that the mind does not stand still. Instead, it will find varied and increasing ways to move away from the object of meditation: the breath. It's the natural tendency of the untrained mind to scatter and be wayward. The key word here is *untrained,* because with practice your mind will begin to settle, especially as you learn to understand distraction.

The only moment that you can ever actually experience is the present moment, and yet we constantly move away it. Often, much of your time is spent skipping around the past, reliving events and interactions with people, sometimes rationalizing or trying to work these events and interactions out after the fact, wishing you had said or done something different than what actually happened. Sometimes you go on sentimental memory journeys. You can get so lost in this activity that the present moment is blotted out. And if these memories have a strong emotional component to them, the implications can be frequent and unintended interruptions that pull you away from mindfulness.

As noted above, in addition to rummaging around in the past, you can get caught up in thoughts about the present, as well as anxious and anticipatory planning for events in the future that may never even materialize. All three directions that your mind will want to take you are all deeply rooted in patterns of habit; you are likely not even aware that your mind is taking you on this ride. I wasn't aware of these little journeys that I would go on, and my active mind would create or review elaborate scenarios. Whichever direction your mind wants to take you, nonjudgmental disengagement is the appropriate response. Notice the thought and drop it, returning your attention to your breath and the present. As you learn this skill, you will begin to recognize when this is happening. As you learn to disengage, your meditation will be even more beneficial, and you will realize the negative affect that the wayward thoughts used to have on you as your life begins to change.

What you are after as you learn to train your mind to drop wayward thoughts is what is known as bare attention. Just as the opening paragraph of this chapter pointed to, the over-complication that the West tries to attach to something as basic as meditation, the power of bare attention lies in its simplicity. The challenge for you, as it was for me because I was obsessed with being productive and having something to show for my time, is that when you are achieving bare attention, it doesn't seem like you are doing anything at best and at worst, it may seem counterproductive, indulgent, or a waste of time. Instead, it is a highly alert and skilled state of mind that few people can actually master because you are neutral, neither adding nor subtracting from your present moment. And as far as productivity is concerned, there is little else that can give you the level of self-care than bare attention meditation.

You can try a bare attention exercise by paying attention to your breath. Start by making sure that you will not be disturbed for about ten minutes, and then sit comfortably. Now pay close, but relaxed attention to your breath as it passes through your nostrils. Feel the sensation of air passing through your nose and over your upper lip. Take natural breaths, without manipulating or altering your breathing in any way. Breathing is an involuntary exercise that goes on throughout your life, but how often do you pay close attention to it?

The quality of the attention that you are paying is important. And it is deliberate that you think of it as paying attention and not, say, concentrating, because the latter creates undue pressure and a rigid focusing, and can make attention difficult to maintain. Rest your attention on your breath in a light and relaxed way, and this will give rise to a natural awareness of the breath coming and going. This simple exercise is remarkable in that a seemingly effortless attention brings you to awareness, and yet achieving this awareness is very difficult for most people. Continue with the relaxed yet focused attention and move it around the breath, notice the natural variation in inhale and exhale, the variation of pressure in one nostril or the other. You will become aware of a number of details, not because you are concentrating, or fixated, or analyzing, but because you have attended to a single act of breath.

And as simple as this all sounds, long before you get to the point of awareness of different aspects of your breath, you will have had invading thoughts, often mere seconds after the breath observation. It is likely that within five breaths, your mind will have wandered. Whether it is trying to figure out where a sound is coming from, or thinking you are crazy for wasting your time sitting idle and paying attention to your breath, or wondering if you are doing it right, this is natural and you just want to mentally drop the thought(s) and return to the breath – without judgment or reaction.

This is what bare attention is about. Whether it was a sound, or your back hurt, or whatever, just note it and move back to breath. You keep the attention bare because you note and move back to breath without analysis, rationalization, elaboration, judgment, or drama, which are the hallmarks of what the mind does with an invading thought if we do not come back to breath. Even if you find yourself in one of these secondary thought processes, returning to breath will restore bare attention. With practice, bare attention becomes a process for dealing with sensory input by acknowledging and letting go, and an effortless check on uncontrolled thought in a gentle manner and without using suppression.

Mindfulness is deceiving in its simplicity, however, and it will take practice to overcome a lifetime of undisciplined thinking. Nevertheless, bare attention makes mindfulness possible, and mindfulness is being present in a knowing way with whatever is happening around you, knowing from moment to moment what is going on, in and around you. Understanding bare attention and mindfulness, you can meditate. Meditation is knowing what is happening while it is happening, no matter what it is. If you are sitting attending to your breath and you are present with your breath, you are meditating because you know what is happening while it is happening. If you are with your breath and thoughts keep invading, or emotions come up, or sounds draw your attention, you are still meditating, so long as you are aware of being drawn away because you still know what is happening in real time. If you doze off or get lost in a daydream, meditation has ended because you no longer know what is happening.

Another pathway to mastering meditation is through the mantra. The word mantra can be broken down into two parts: *man*, which means mind, and *tra*, which means transport or vehicle. In other words, a mantra is an instrument of the mind – a powerful sound, word, words, or vibration that you can use to enter a deep state of meditation. Practically speaking, a mantra gives the mind something to focus on. Mantra recitation, which is called japa or *muttering* in Sanskrit, has been an important aspect of yoga practice since Vedic times. It consists of the repetition of the same mantra, which can be composed of a single syllable like *om* or *ang*, or a string of mantric sounds like *om namah shivaya*. Other sample mantras include *om namo Narayana, om miyoho renge kyo* and *ang sang weha guru.*

Today there are YouTube videos with an endless array of themes for meditation and meditation phone apps like Head-space that give the mind something to latch onto instead of the breath. While traditional, breath-based meditation is the solid foundation on which I learned, using electronic medi-tation aids are an easier way in for many people who would have otherwise given up. But fair warning, even with noise in your ears to occupy your mind or a mantra to silently chant, there will still be invading thoughts that you will need to learn to contend with. There is no magic bullet, and some effort is required on your part to master mindfulness.

When I was in the middle of my fight with cancer compounded by the emotional anguish of my then-wife's infidelity, my primary care physician diagnosed me with post-traumatic stress disorder. I didn't like the term *disorder* because I knew it was episodic and not a long-term condi-tion. Was I under stress? You betcha. But anyone in similar conditions would be, too. He prescribed pills for me. I read the side effects on the side of the box and discovered that one of the many side effects was the potential to want to commit suicide. I refused to take them and told the doctor that I was fighting for my life and I would be damned if I was going to take something that might make me want to kill myself. I already crossed that Rubicon and instead had embraced a reason to live (see Chapter 9). But this experience is one of several that led me to meditation and eventually to the prac-tice of hypnotherapy.

I am certified in hypnotherapy for post-traumatic stress disorder clients who, like cancer clients, experience hyper-vigilance that results in over-active self-talk. The first thing I do is teach them mindfulness and meditation, and then I anchor these processes with hypnotherapy. I had a client, Amy, who was struggling with the loss of her parents and became distraught when she was steamrolled by her siblings, who in the absence of clear direction in the will took everything. This left my client with nothing but anxiety, stress, and fear accompanied by mild paranoia. She couldn't work and could barely function. When I taught her to meditate, she regained perspective, quieted her mind, and was able to land another job and get back on her feet.

The power of meditation is immeasurable. I listed meditation first among the seven steps because getting control of your mind and your thoughts is really the first step of taking charge of your health.

Exercise: Bare Attention

1. Find a private place where you will not be disturbed.

2. Sit on a comfortable seat with your back straight.

3. Close your eyes, relax, and place your attention on your breath.

4. Stay observant of all that comes to your awareness, whatever it might be. If thoughts invade, disengage as soon as you notice and return to breath.

5. Try to get to five minutes straight. Then try two more five-minute stretches.

6. Check in on yourself throughout the day to see if you are being mindful – do you know what you are doing while you are doing it? The true value of meditation is to train ourselves to be ever mindful and present.

7. Continue this exercise every day for a week. See if you can work your way to 30 minutes.

Exercise: Staying Present

1. Repeat steps 1-3 above.

2. For the first 10 minutes of the session, relax and practice bare attention.

3. Take a short, 30-second break and relax the body while you look off into space or out a window.

4. Return to practicing bare attention.

5. Now each time your mind wanders away from breath, make note where it went. Past thoughts? Present fantasizing or thinking? Future planning? What triggered the invading thought? A sound, a sensation? Spontaneous? A returning thought, or a new one? Some other reason?

CHAPTER 4
EAT TO LIVE

*"What lies behind us and what lies before us are
tiny matters compared to what lies within us."*
Ralph Waldo Emerson*

There seems to be some controversy over the attribution of the quote above. I won't go into the sordid details of the discussion over precisely where the words originated, rather I'll just go with my favorite, Emerson. And let's not get caught up in the fairly oblique philosophical reference of *what lies inside* and whether it can appropriately be applied to food, because it could just as likely apply to the next chapter on spirituality, although I would argue that you need to take an almost spiritual approach to what you feed your body.

Today in the United States, we have an amazingly efficient food production process that delivers to a store nearby a vast array of food choices unmatched in the world. There are affordable prepared food options on every street corner and from nearly all ethnic origins. The government, after some high-profile food preparation and packaging horror stories over a hundred years ago, has a fairly vast and detailed regulatory regime for food safety, requiring the labeling of contents and the disclosure of the relative nutrient values of what it has determined to be the average daily consumption requirement of various ingredients.

In fact, the United States Food and Drug Administration (USFDA) Food Safety Modernization Act (FSMA), the most sweeping reform of our food safety laws in more than 70 years, was signed into law by President Obama on January 4, 2011. It aims to ensure the US food supply is safe by shifting the focus from responding to contamination, to preventing it. Foodborne illness is a significant burden, says the FDA, in that about 48 million (1 in 6 Americans) get sick each year; 128,000 are hospitalized; 3,000 die; and young and immune-compromised individuals are more susceptible. For them, including infants and children, pregnant women, older individuals, and those on chemotherapy, foodborne illness is not just a stomachache, it can cause life-long chronic diseases like arthritis and kidney failure.

Good news that the government is at work enacting laws to protect us, right? But wait a minute, we have had a pretty rigorous regulatory regime for some time, and yet, nearly 50 million Americans get sick from food every year? At the same time, because there is a 30 to 40 percent waste factor for food, government and industry are both concerned about increasing food shelf life, and this leads to a greater use of chemical preservatives. The packaging may be prescribed and the labeling required, but do you really know what the impacts of some of those preservative ingredients are?

Alright, so food is cheap and plentiful, and the government has an ever-increasing regulatory oversight presence looking out for you. You're busy and you don't like to cook, can't you just take advantage of the quick and easy food that seems to be readily at your fingertips? The government is watching, and those preservative chemicals would not be allowed into our food if they were dangerous, and you know processed food has less nutritional value than fresh food, but if you eat mostly from the four food groups, won't you be alright?

Now that you have learned to meditate in the last chapter, I encourage you to sit with that thinking and see how it makes you feel. Detachment from how and what we eat, and a pattern of eating what is loosely referred to as the *Western* diet, is arguably the foundation for illness, chronic illness, and even disease.

In a 2005 American Society for Clinical Nutrition study titled *Origins and evolution of the Western diet: health implications for the 21st century*, researchers noted that there was growing awareness that the profound changes in the human environment, such as diet and other lifestyle conditions that began with the introduction of agriculture and animal husbandry approximately 10,000 years ago, occurred too recently on an evolutionary time scale for the human genome to adjust. As the nutritional, cultural, and activity patterns of contemporary Western populations developed, our ancient, genetically determined biology has not evolved on pace, and this has resulted in the emergence of many of what are referred to as the *diseases of civilization*. Of particular significance, food staples and food-processing procedures introduced during the industrial period have fundamentally altered seven crucial nutritional characteristics of ancestral human diets: 1) glycemic load, 2) fatty acid composition, 3) macronutrient composition, 4) micronutrient density, 5) acid-base balance, 6) sodium-potassium ratio, and 7) fiber content. The research pointed to the notion that the evolutionary collision of our ancient genome with the nutritional qualities of recently introduced foods may underlie many of the chronic diseases of Western civilization.

The study went on to report that in the United States, chronic illnesses and health problems either in whole, or in part attributable to diet, represent a serious threat to public health. Sixty percent of adults older than 20 are either overweight or obese, and the estimated number of deaths attributable to obesity is 280,184 per year. More than 64 million have cardiovascular disease, which represents the leading cause of mortality (38.5 percent of all deaths). Fifty million Americans are hypertensive; 11 million have type 2 diabetes, and 37 million adults maintain high-risk cholesterol concentrations. In postmenopausal women over 50, 7.2 percent have osteoporosis and 39.6 percent have osteopenia. Osteoporotic hip fractures are associated with a 20 percent excess mortality in the year after fracture. *Cancer is the second leading cause of death (25 percent of all deaths), and an estimated one-third of all cancer deaths are due to nutritional factors, including obesity.*

That the human genome was unprepared for the rapid transformation of the modern human diet is pretty obvious if you consider how quickly life has changed in the last 150 years; but technology is accelerating the level and extent of processing and portends larger scale impacts on health if you do not pay active attention to what you consume. Researchers have found that highly processed food purchases are a dominant and growing part of purchasing patterns among Americans, and are likely to have higher saturated fat, sugar, and sodium content compared with less-processed foods.

As the body of research grows, diet has been gaining attention as a potential contributor to the increase in immune-related diseases. As previously noted, the Western diet is characterized by an over-consumption of refined sugars, salt, and saturated fat. The impacts and mechanisms of harm for our over-indulgence in sugar, salt, and fat, and the impacts of artificial sweeteners, gluten, and genetically modified foods are becoming clear. The dietary impact on the gut microbiome and our poor dietary choices are being encoded into our gut and our genes (albeit slowly), and are passed to our offspring. While today's modern diet may provide beneficial protection from micro- and macronutrient deficiencies, our overabundance of calories and the macronutrients that compose our diet may all lead to increased inflammation, reduced control of infection, increased rates of cancer, and increased risk for allergic and auto-inflammatory disease.

This all seems pretty obvious when you think about it. The problem is that we don't think much about it. Busy schedules, convenience, and sometimes manipulation by advertising, or even the increased sugar content of virtually every processed food sends you into an auto-pilot action toward a diet that can kill you. What if I told you that there was another way to think about food? Before your diagnosis, you may have been vaguely aware of the debate over food that we have just been highlighting, but you now have a stake in seeing food differently.

The second important action I took when faced with my cancer challenge was to change the way I looked at food. The yogi who taught me to meditate had a thing or two to teach me about food.

In Hindu philosophy including yoga, Ayurveda (Indian medicine), and martial arts, *prana* is cosmic energy that permeates the Universe. Prana is often referred to as the *life force*. In the physical body, we have two types of energies: prana, and mind or consciousness. This means that in every organ of the body there should be two channels supplying energy. Modern physiology describes two types of nervous systems, the sympathetic and the parasympathetic, and these two nervous systems are interconnected in each and every organ of the body. You can think of the two, two-track systems as corollaries.

In the context of food, pranic life force requires that the food you consume be close to where it originated. The closer the food from where it was grown or raised, the more life force it contains. Conversely, the further from production and more processed, the less the life force, or nutritional value of the food.

It is time to begin making a deliberate and conscious decision to eat food that has greater life force, and less sugar and fat, fewer preservatives. In short, eating from an energetic and cellular approach. Let's go back and take a page out of the Western medicine book of materialism. The cells of the food you eat get broken down and turned into the cells of your body. We literally *are* what we eat!

Returning to Dr. Turner's *Radical Remission*, she points out that the Greek physician known as the founder of modern medicine, Hippocrates, believed that food has the power to heal the body. She went on to lament her findings that medical students receive only one week of instruction on nutrition in the whole four years of medical school. Nevertheless, she found that among those she studied who healed from cancer, the majority tended to make the same four dietary changes: significantly reducing or eliminating sugar, meat, dairy, and processed foods; greatly increasing consumption of fruits and vegetables; eating organic foods; and drinking filtered and alkaline water.

Again, you shouldn't be too surprised by the foregoing list, these are the usual suspects of the Western diet that need to be reduced or eliminated. For example, not only does sugar intake increase your glycemic index and lead to poor health that can turn quickly to disease, sugar (glucose) is known to be metabolized by cancer cells at a much faster rate than normal cells. This fact is used in the positron emission tomography (PET) scan process in which you drink glucose and the scanner highlights the areas of the body that are metabolizing sugar the fastest.

Dairy products are packed with hormones and proteins to make a baby calf grow and the main protein in milk, casein, like sugar, feeds cancer cells. Never mind that dairy products contain unhealthy chemicals like growth hormone and antibiotics and that cows are fed corn because it's cheap, dairy products have unhealthy amounts of omega-6 fats, which have been linked to cancer. But eating can be emotional. I used to eat large amounts of ice cream even though it caused gastric distress. Today, with the availability of almond milk, I had reduced my dairy intake to small amounts of cheese, because let's face it, who can live without cheese? Humor aside, eventually I even eliminated cheese from my diet.

The correlation between cancer and high intake of red meat has been demonstrated in numerous studies and many of the same issues with dairy, like hormones and omega-6 fats, combine with long digestion cycles to argue against more than minimal, if any, red meat consumption. Studies have also shown that red meat consumption promotes inflammation, which has a strong cancer link. Red meat was a harder thing to give up, as I did love a good steak. The kicker for me was when I realized how long it sits in your gut digesting when I lost 10 pounds after having had a colonoscopy. I went from eating beef a couple times a month to not at all, because in addition to the terrible health effects, I felt sluggish after doing so. Eventually, I gave it up altogether and am heathier for it.

Finally, processed or refined foods are *no bueno* because they are very high on the glycemic index, which means that their carbohydrates are quickly turned into glucose, which as noted is cancer jet-fuel. So, bread, pasta, and grains should be reduced or eliminated, and instead whole grains like brown rice, quinoa, wheat berries, whole oats, and barley should be consumed, which have more dietary fiber and vitamins, anyway.

Higher amounts of fresh fruits and vegetables give a human body everything it needs from vitamins and minerals to fiber, protein, and even good fats. Studies have even shown that many fruits and vegetables have anti-cancer properties. Whole books have been written on the benefits of cruciferous vegetables like broccoli, cauliflower, and cabbage as well as allium vegetables like onions and garlic as potent cancer-fighting foods. Juicing your fruits and vegetables is a nutritious way to get the raw, unmitigated benefits from these super foods. This is the domain of prana – life force.

In addition to life force, easily digestible foods give your organs the chance to cleanse at night instead of being tied up by digestion, so if you do not eat late and eat a mostly plant-based diet, your organs cleanse, releasing toxins. You sleep better, too.

Taking it a step further, making sure your fruits and vegetables are organically grown will help you detox from the accumulation of toxins and pesticides that collect in your body from environmental exposure. When you consider that a recent study in the *Annals of Internal Medicine* titled, *Are Organic Foods Safer or Healthier than Conventional Alternatives? A Systematic Review*, found that organic food is 30 percent less likely to contain pesticides, it should be a no-brainer.

Finally, since we are 70 percent water in our physical make up, staying hydrated is critical to good health, and drinking filtered water is going to shield you from chlorine, fluoride, and heavy metals that can be present in tap water. A filtration system that can also increase alkalinity will reduce the acidic environment that cancer likes. Alkaline antioxidant water has great efficacy in health maintenance, providing better hydration, and the effect of alkalization and antioxidants is well established. And remember the seven crucial nutritional characteristics of ancestral human diets addressed the acid-base balance. Alkaline water should play a critical role for you in maintaining a healthy balance between acidity and alkalinity.

There are many benefits to eating well, and we just looked at some consistent dietary changes that studied survivors undertook, but can diet alone prevent certain cancers from returning? There is strong evidence that a plant-based diet cuts the risk of cancer overall, and many studies have shown that people who eat diets rich in fruits and vegetables and sparse in meat and animal fat have lower rates of some cancers, including lung, breast, colon, and stomach cancers.

On the way to healing and recovery, it is really important to remember when you are developing new habits and strategies that plant foods contain antioxidants such as beta-carotene, lycopene, and vitamins A, C, and E, which protect the cells from free radicals – unstable molecules that damage healthy cells and are linked to aging and disease. Phytochemicals, also found in fruits, vegetables, legumes, and grains, are compounds that may thwart the action of carcinogens and aid cells in blocking the development or recurrence of cancer.

Further, there is evidence that being overweight, which is a risk factor for numerous types of cancer, also increases the chance of recurrence and lowers odds for survival. Research has shown that women who gain more than 13 pounds during treatment for early-stage breast cancer are 1.5 times more likely to experience a cancer recurrence. Studies show that for men who have had prostate cancer, being overweight or obese raises the chances that their cancer will recur, spread, or lead to death. These statistics argue strenuously for the importance of radically changing your diet.

The various treatments have varying effects. For example, some people lose weight because chemotherapy and radiation side effects such as nausea, taste changes, and loss of appetite make eating difficult. Further, therapeutic effects can impair the absorption of nutrients. Conversely, some people may put on pounds from medications, reduced activity, or emotional and stress-related eating.

As a cancer survivor, you should consider the following guidelines for a healthy diet:

You should eat a minimum of five servings of fruits and vegetables a day. Use plant-based seasonings like parsley and my favorites, turmeric and cardamom. As noted above, eat whole grains including high-fiber breads and cereals, including brown rice, barley, bulgur, and oats; avoid refined foods, such as donuts and white bread, and those high in sugar.

Plants have all the protein you will need, but if you must eat meat, choose lean protein. Stick to fish, poultry, and even try tofu. The point is to limit red meat and processed meats, and keep dairy low fat if you consume it at all. Plan for a variety of foods and create a balanced plate that is half cooked or raw vegetables, a quarter lean protein (chicken, fish, lean meat, or dairy), and a quarter whole grains. I have eliminated meat altogether and you should consider it, too.

You should have salmon, sardines, and tuna at least twice a week, as the fats in these fish are the heart-healthy omega-3 fats; other sources of these fats include walnuts and flaxseeds. But even fish is now questionable as mercury and other biocumulative chemicals contaminate much of the commercially available seafood.

Limit alcohol consumption. Alcohol has been linked to cancer risk. Men should have no more than two drinks a day; women should have no more than one drink.

Eat foods high in vitamin D. These include salmon, sardines, fortified orange juice, milk, and fortified cereal. Research suggests that vitamin D, which also comes from sun exposure, prevents cancer and may decrease the risk of recurrence and improve survival.

In the end, eating has such an emotional context, and sugar is right there in the middle of it. Eating habits have formed over years and are often driven by convenience and/or necessity. Even when your life depends on changing your eating habits, many people still struggle. This is why hypnotherapy is such an integral element of my practice and a tool in helping people make these seven critical changes in their behavior when faced with the challenge of cancer.

My client, Diana, knew that she immediately needed to address her sugar issues after her diagnosis. After a solid hypnotherapy session on overcoming sugar cravings, she returned to tell me she had fallen off the wagon and binged on sweets. In the cognitive interview before we went back into hypnosis, I decided to explore the emotional aspect of her sweet tooth. She had told me in the original interview that her mother had passed away several years before, and we discussed whether she had dealt conclusively with the stages of loss. She believed she had, but now I wasn't so sure.

I asked her if her mother had baked for her as a child. She answered that she had. As a child, her mother always had cookies and cakes and other sweet baked goods that they baked together, and that the smell of the kitchen while baking brought up deep emotions for her. It turns out that the anniversary of her mother's passing was approaching. Diana always put on a celebration of life for her, and it was coming up. Instead of doing another session on sugar, we did a session on coping with the stages of loss, and the sugar issue went away.

Eating to live is not always easy, and changing behavior is hard. Borrowing from the computer world, *garbage in, garbage out*. But approaching it as behavioral change is so important, and here is why. Do you know why so many diets do not work? It is because people change their eating behavior based on the latest and greatest diet and lose weight. Then, they go back to their *normal* eating behavior and wonder why they put the weight back on and then some. The *then some* comes about because the return to the *normal* diet is undertaken with a vengeance after the diet and weight loss left you wanting. To be successful at eating to live, you must approach it in a sustainable manner, and you really need to support the behavioral change with the powerful tool of hypnotherapy to overcome the historical, emotional, and subconscious factors that influence your eating habits.

CHAPTER 5

THE ONLY WAY IS THROUGH SPIRIT

"All major religious traditions carry basically the same message, that is love, compassion and forgiveness … the important thing is they should be part of our daily lives."

Dalai Lama

Deepening spirituality. It is as important as each of the other steps to healing and recovery, but it is a hot potato if ever there was one. People have fought and died over the subject, countries have gone to war. No matter which direction you turn to cover the topic, someone is likely to be offended, so I am going to do my best eggshell walk. I just ask that you keep an open mind and understand the importance of nurturing your spirit and connecting to a divine spirit that is bigger than you, has as its nature unconditional love, and is characterized by forgiveness and gratitude.

Every fall for ten years, I would pull my kids out of school and vacation in Hawaii for two weeks. We went in the fall because, as a lobbyist, when the legislature was in session and my clients could potentially be affected by the plenary power of the legislators, I had to be there standing guard. In 2008, as we were preparing for our annual Hawaiian vacation, I went by the bank where I had my personal and business accounts to take care of some transactions before leaving. As I walked up the pedestrian K Street in Sacramento, I saw a scene right out of *It's a Wonderful Life*, where there was a run on the Savings and Loan, and George Bailey saved the day by giving people just enough money to tide them over from his own savings. There were people lined up at Washington Mutual, and the line was pouring out into the street. The bank manager, who I had known for some time, pleaded with me not to remove all of my holdings. I hedged and only moved half, moving the other half to Bank of America because they weren't selling or panicking, they were buying!

And off to Hawaii I went. But it was very difficult to relax. Our country's financial institutions were in meltdown. Presidential candidates suspended their campaigns to return to Washington to work on legislation. My bank, Washington Mutual, failed and was purchased by Chase. They were uncertain times.

I was an adventure traveler and was usually off on activities like hiking, golfing, and snorkeling, not one to sit around the pool and read. But this year, I had brought a book that I had been meaning to read, thinking that the flight and airport time would give me a chance to wade in. The book was *Zen and Birds of Appetite*, by Thomas Merton, and it was a collection of essays between Merton, a Catholic priest, and

D. T. Suzuki, a Zen Buddhist, comparing and contrasting Christianity and Zen Buddhism. As it turns out, it was a perfect read for the trying times that were threatening to completely overshadow my vacation.

Each page was filled with deep concepts and needed to be read twice, and sometimes three times, for proper understanding. Even then, further reflection followed in the twilight before sleep and over morning coffee. Consider the following passage:

> *"Both Christianity and Buddhism show that suffering remains inexplicable, most of all for the man who attempts to explain it in order to evade it, or who thinks explanation itself is an escape. Suffering is not a 'problem' as if it were something we could stand outside of and control. Suffering, as both Christianity and Buddhism see, each in its own way, is part of our very ego-identity and empirical existence, and the only thing to do about it is to plunge right into the middle of contradiction and confusion in order to be transformed by what Zen calls' the great death' and Christianity calls' dying and rising with Christ.'"*

To dive into a deep and meaningful theological exploration of life and its meaning was a perfect foil for the crazy period we were living through, and it gave me context for life. To consider if the basic teachings of Buddhism on ignorance, deliverance and enlightenment are really life-denying, or rather the same kind of life-affirming liberation that we find in the redemption, the Gift of the Spirit, were questions that helped me transcend the political chaos ever so briefly. And to contemplate the notion that Zen emptiness is not the emptiness of nothingness, but the emptiness of fullness, in which there is no gain, no loss, no increase, no decrease and is expressed as zero equals infinity, gave me a great deal of comfort because, although I didn't know it at the time, it introduced me to a departure from duality and toward singularity, and ultimately gave me enough peace to enjoy my vacation.

Three years later, I was diagnosed with cancer. One of my first acts was to dig up my copy of *Zen and the Birds of Appetite*. I had often thought of the mind-expanding exercise reading that book had been and the spiritual growth I experienced as a result of reading it. The author's note at the beginning was a hauntingly poignant description of Zen as only available to those with the right perspective, and I knew that I desperately needed perspective.

> *"Where there is clarion lying, meat eating birds circle and descend. Life and death are two. The living attack the dead, to their own profit. The dead lose nothing by it. They gain, too, by being disposed of. Or they seem to, if you must think in terms of gain and loss. Do you then approach the study of Zen with the idea that there is something to be gained by it? This question is not intended as an implicit accusation. But it is, nevertheless, a serious question. Where there is a lot of fuss about*

spirituality, enlightenment ... it is often because there are buzzards hovering around a corpse. This hovering, this circling, this descending, this celebration of victory, are not what is meant by the Study of Zen – even though they may be a highly useful exercise in other contexts. And they enrich the birds of appetite.

"Zen enriches no one. There is no body to be found. The birds may come and circle for a while in the place that it is thought to be. But they soon go elsewhere. When they are gone, the 'nothing,' the 'no-body' that was there, suddenly appears. That is Zen. It was there all the time but the scavengers missed it, because it was not their kind of prey."

Spirituality is there for you, but you must have eyes to see it. If not, you will hover and circle over the place you think it to be, but will not find it. This is one of the most profound passages that I have ever read. Now that you have read it, let's look at what deepening your spirituality looks like, for you.

So often any discussion of spirituality turns – if not immediately then fairly quickly – to religion. As a result, and because people generally have deeply held beliefs or conversely, aversions to religion, the conversation either ends, or turns heated. In her book, *Anatomy of the Spirit*, Carolyn Myss writes that from her very first medical intuition experiences, she knew they were about the human *spirit*. These were physical problems and she used energy terms to describe them to others, because she didn't want to evoke religious connotations or deeply held fears about someone's relationship with God. *Energy* is a value neutral word, and she had found that it was much easier and usually better received to tell someone their energy was depleted, rather than telling them that their spirit was toxic.

She goes on to detail that her evolution toward the acceptance and incorporation of the spiritual implications of illness and the impetus for her book was her realization while teaching a workshop on energy that the seven chakras, or energy centers, in the body aligned with the seven sacraments of Christianity, as well as the seven teachings of the Kabbalah. What's more, as she dove into the correlations, she found that spirituality is far more than an emotional and psychological need, it's an essential biological need, and our energy, spirit, and personal power are of the same force.

Myss's epiphany was an *aha* moment for me, too. We have a biological need for spirituality and our energy, spirit and personal power are of the same force. To understand this is to understand the root of your personal power. I have seen relatives and clients who become angry at *God* for their sickness or the sickness of loved ones, and I just want to share that this response is a power-robbing emotional response. Perspective and maintaining perspective are so very critical to moving beyond coping and into healing and recovery.

Whether you are religious and attend a church, synagogue, mosque or temple; or a deist who believes in a divine being but doesn't attend church; an agnostic; or an atheist, you cannot ignore the universal message that we have a biological need to foster spirituality, and any healing that takes place will come with nurturing a spiritual path. If you have a priest, a pastor, a rabbi, a mullah, or a rishi, then you have someone to turn to for guidance and a community of spiritual support, and I encourage you to use this framework to deepen your spirituality. If you are not someone with a spiritual framework, let the following guide you to discovery. It really is our life's purpose to nurture and understand our spirit, and our health and well-being depend on it. Every thought, belief, and memory we have translates into a positive or negative impact on our spirit.

I once saw Wayne Dyer speak at a Hay House event. He was supposed to speak for an hour on the Friday night opening of the event, from 8:00 p.m. to 9:00 p.m. He spoke from 8:00 p.m. to 11:00 p.m., and no one left early. I loved the way he described his approach to spirituality. He said we are not earthbound beings having periodic spiritual experiences; we are spiritual beings living a temporary earthbound existence. Wayne said he believed in God, but he said he wanted to reach the widest possible audience so he came to refer to the divine as source energy. It is from source energy that we come when we are born, and it is to source energy that we return when we die. Our spirit is animated by that source energy, as is everyone else's, which is why we need to have unconditional love for our fellow humans because they are all perfect little drops of God, or source. The challenge is that we develop an ego that separates us from source and each other, emphasizing the duality of life. Nevertheless, he was encouraging and optimistic in that he believed that at any time we could connect with the divine mind.

We learn about the world through opposites: night and day, light and dark, good and bad, love and hate. This duality leads us to separate ourselves from others and from the divine, but our goal and a biological need is to reconnect with the divine and live a spiritual life. When you are able to connect to the divine and have a spiritual experience, it can have an emotional impact, almost like a warm, fuzzy feeling that connects the physical and emotional aspects of the body. And while everyone is different and one person may respond to a deep meditation and another to a prayer circle, the important thing is to find what speaks to you spiritually and practice it daily so that you can experience that peaceful spiritual energy on a regular and ongoing basis.

There is an ancient proverb that suggests that the doctor dresses the wound and God heals it. It is our willingness to commune with the divine spirit that harnesses the same creative intelligence that assembled your parts and jump-started your heart, and applies it to your healing. There is another saying that I am fond of that goes something like this: Prayer is you talking to God; meditation is God answering.

The power of prayer cannot be overestimated. Do you pray? Most people say a prayer when they are confronted with an emergency, trouble, danger or illness, or at the behest of someone else facing similar difficulties. These are known as petition prayers and can be likened to throwing up a Hail Mary, as in the desperate downfield pass in football, not as part of the Catholic rosary. For prayer to be effective, it has to be consistent. If you want the divine to show up, you need to show up for the divine on a regular and ongoing basis.

Having a consistent prayer practice will make prayer easier and more meaningful in those troubled times when you are in distress and may have difficulty thinking clearly.

Joseph Murphy, in his book, *The Power of Your Subconscious Mind*, refers to scientific prayer, which he says occurs when your conscious mind and subconscious mind work together in unison. Even Western medicine has weighed in on the topic of prayer. A WebMD article from 2004 titled, *Can Prayer Heal*, cited Dr. Mitchell Krucoff, a cardiovascular specialist at Duke University Medical School, who has been studying prayer and spirituality since 1996 and practicing it much longer in his patient care. Dr. Krucoff noted that early studies of the healing powers of prayer were small and often flawed. Some were in the form of anecdotal reports, with descriptions of miracles in patients with cancer, pain syndromes, and heart disease. He said that we're now beginning to see systematic investigations, clinical research as well as position statements from professional societies supporting this research, federal subsidies from the National Institute for Health, funding from Congress, and all of these studies, all the reports, are remarkably consistent in suggesting the potential measurable health benefit associated with prayer or spiritual interventions.

The article went on to note Harvard scientist Herbert Benson, M.D., who for 30 years has conducted his own studies on prayer and meditation. All forms of prayer, he says, *evoke a relaxation response that quells stress, quiets the body, and promotes healing.*

Benson has documented on MRI brain scans the physical changes that take place in the body when someone meditates or prays. When combined with recent research from the University of Pennsylvania, what emerges is a picture of complex brain activity wherein everything registers as emotionally significant, perhaps responsible for the sense of awe and quiet that many feel. The body becomes more relaxed and physiological activity becomes more evenly regulated.

In the end, to deepen your spiritual awareness, you first need to become more mindful of both your inner and outer worlds. Spiritual awareness is the recognition and attention to the fact that you are but a part of a much greater reality than you can perceive with your five senses. As simple as this sounds, the problem is like the Western medicine description of meditation in Chapter 3, our uber-developed, logical brains get in the way of the *knowing* of this greater reality that is beyond logic.

You just need a little humble wisdom to know you're only a part of a greater divinity. Deep and meaningful spiritual awareness doesn't require a middle man between you and the Divine, it just requires you to think and believe beyond you and your five senses. My journey through cancer led me to a deep embrace of spirituality. Up to this point in my life, I had been a surveyor. I wasn't raised with religion, and when I got to college, I dove into world religions, read widely among the greatest texts, and took many classes as part of my philosophy minor. But this was arm's-length spirituality. I didn't join or subscribe to any world religion or world view, although I respected the best attributes of all that I studied.

As a political science major, I had read extensively on the founding fathers and particularly liked what Thomas Jefferson referred to as Deism, the belief in a divine creator who shed providence with an invisible hand. I settled safely in there, but it required little, if anything, of me and as a result yielded little, if any real spirituality. But it sounded cool.

My survey continued after college and into my thirties. I studied Buddhism while trekking in Nepal, I read the Koran. What I came to realize when I got sick was that while all of these efforts were no doubt intellectually enriching, they were external; I needed to internalize my spirituality and really embrace the tenets of a deepened, personal spirituality. So, in my meditation I imagined Jesus in my heart center and I emanated love to everyone in my life and forgiveness to all, even those who I previously could not have found my way to forgive. I meditated to a mantra of love, kindness, gratitude, and forgiveness. I found my way to Hay House, broadened my readings, and attended one of their *I Can Do It* conferences. And I began to pray. Not the petition prayers that we discussed above. A deep, meaningful conversation with the Divine. And I showed up every day.

Ultimately, whether you follow a particular religion or not, here are a few tips to help you cultivate deeper spiritual awareness and strengthen your connection with the Divine.

Practice radical forgiveness; embrace total gratitude; give unconditional love; and do these things on a daily basis.

CHAPTER 6
POWER BEYOND MEASURE

*"As you sow in your subconscious mind, so shall you
reap in your body and your environment."*
Joseph Murphy

In Chapter 2, you got a look at the difference between the brain and the mind, but now it is time to talk about a similar, but different cerebral bifurcation: conscious versus subconscious mind.

The conscious mind is the part of your mind that is responsible for logic, analysis, decision-making, reasoning, and will power. If I asked you to add numbers together, it's your conscious mind that is going to be used to perform that addition.

The conscious mind also controls all the actions that you do on purpose, or with intention, while being conscious. For example, when you decide to take any voluntary action like moving your hand or leg, it is done by the conscious mind. Whenever you are aware of the thing you're doing, you can be sure that you are doing it by your conscious mind. If there is a cup of tea beside you and you decide to take a sip, then this process will be done by your conscious mind because you are completely conscious while doing it.

The subconscious mind is the part of your mind responsible for all of your *involuntary* actions. For example, your breathing and heartbeats are controlled by your subconscious mind. If, beginning to meditate, you started to control your breath on intention, then know that your conscious mind took charge. Conversely, if you were breathing without being conscious of the breathing process, then know that your subconscious mind is in charge. Simplified, but illustrative. It controls the circulation of your blood, your digestion, and elimination. In short, your subconscious mind controls all of the vital processes and functions of your body.

Your subconscious operates on what is referred to as the *homeostatic* impulse. And just as it keeps you breathing regularly and keeps your heart beating at a certain rate, it keeps your body temperature at 98.6 degrees. Through your autonomic nervous system, it maintains a balance among the hundreds of chemicals in your billions of cells so that your entire physical body functions in complete harmony when operating properly. Your subconscious mind also practices homeostasis in your mental realm by keeping you thinking and acting consistently with how you have acted in the past and according to your established belief patterns.

Your emotions are also controlled by your subconscious mind. That's why you sometimes might feel afraid, anxious, or down without actually *wanting* to experience such a feeling. The subconscious mind never sleeps and never rests.

When the conscious mind is asleep, the subconscious is busy processing the input of your senses and ciphering this input by literal and symbolic interpretation through your system of beliefs in the form of dreams.

The subconscious is a goal machine. If you deliberately and intentionally set out your goals for something that you want to achieve every night before you fall asleep through prayer, meditation, and/or journaling, you will be amazed that forces within you will be released to deliver you to your desired result. It is the wellspring of inspiration, of art and creation. When it is said that we only fully use a fraction of our brain, it is the hugely untapped subconscious that is the underutilized, yet powerful potential portion being referred to.

Conversely, and just as the nocebo was to the placebo, if you think destructively or negatively, destructive emotions are generated so that they must find an outlet, and it is often tension, anxiety, ulcers, or other physical conditions, including disease (dis-ease), that manifest. Remember the discussion about self-talk: it is the subconscious that is listening. The subconscious mind does not differentiate between right and wrong; it comprehends in knowns and unknowns.

Your subconscious mind is like a huge memory bank. Its capacity is virtually unlimited. It permanently stores everything that ever happens to you. It is estimated that by the time you turn 21, you've already permanently stored more than one hundred times the contents of the entire *Encyclopedia Britannica*. It is the second filter in a three-filter system:

the senses are the first filter, bringing in information from the overwhelming world around you; the subconscious is the second filter that measures the information against your programming and belief system; and the third filter is the conscious mind that decides what to think about the information after it has been reduced to a manageable input from the first two filters.

The function of your subconscious mind is to ensure that you respond exactly the way you are programmed. Your subconscious mind makes everything you say and do fit a pattern consistent with your self-concept, your *programming*. As noted, your subconscious mind is subjective, it does not think or reason independently.

Joseph Murphy, in *The Power of Your Subconscious Mind*, warns to only give your subconscious suggestions that heal, bless, elevate, and inspire, because your subconscious mind cannot take a joke and instead takes you at your word. The book is a wealth of understanding and direction for the care and feeding of your subconscious mind. Consider that the law of the subconscious mind *works for good and bad ideas alike. This law, when applied in a negative way, is the cause of failure, frustration, and unhappiness. However, when your habitual thinking is harmonious and constructive, you experience perfect health, success, and prosperity.* Murphy suggests that infinite power is at our fingertips if we can master what he calls *scientific prayer*, which he describes as the harmonious interaction of the conscious and subconscious, scientifically directed toward a specific purpose.

Up to this point, we have looked at the subconscious as separate from the conscious and as a repository of everything we have ever experienced, which has become the basis for our programming. We have also looked at the power of the subconscious and the amazing things we can do with concerted action and persistence, as well as how negative thoughts can bring about equally negative outcomes. Let's now look at how that programming came about.

All of your current beliefs around self-worth, health, money, love, relationships, fear, success, happiness, and every other attitude or belief are pretty much the same beliefs you had when you were 10 years old. I know, sounds unbelievable, but it is true. The reason is that most of your subconscious programming happened between the ages of 0-8, and unless you have worked specifically on changing those beliefs, they continue to be your programming today. As we have seen, subconscious beliefs are at your core, and your subconscious mind is 90 percent of who you are.

The subconscious mind's function is to store and recall memory forever, so you don't have to keep relearning the same things every day. It's where the blueprint of all your habits, beliefs, memories, learning, and physiological processes are held, so you can easily navigate your world and stay consistent with your programmed identity.

The reason our programming from childhood is so long-lasting is that between the ages of 0-8, we are essentially in a hypnotic, trance-like state and absorbing everything around us. Children are subconsciously picking up and storing everything that the adults around them are doing, feeling, and saying in order to figure out how to navigate their own world. Parents, teachers, friends, even television all play a role in our programming. Our sense of identity is contingent upon our early subconscious programming.

Your subconscious blueprint was downloaded through three avenues: verbal programming, which happened when you heard adults speaking to each other or to you when you were growing up, and if something was repeated enough times it got stored in your subconscious memory; modeling, which was when you saw how your parents and other adults around you behaved, their actions and reactions to different situations and people influenced your understanding of how to engage with the world; and specific experiences you had while growing up that impacted your learning process. Everything that happened in your childhood and early adulthood taught you how to survive, live, and thrive.

Not all of your exposure fell into the thrive category, however, and some of the programming led to the development of bad habits, self-limiting beliefs, and distorted perceptions. There are a couple tools for behavioral change and habit control. We already looked at one: mindfulness and meditation. Meditation as a proactive measure is a really great tool to increase your self-awareness and change your thinking habits. Slowing down, even for just five minutes per day, has tremendous benefits for your mind and body. Just by sitting still and focusing on your breath, you are able to increase self-awareness and change your internal state, which makes it more likely that your subconscious will accept the changes you are trying to make.

The other is hypnosis, which is simply a deep state of relaxation and focused attention where it is possible to give suggestions to your subconscious mind to make changes. Going into a hypnotic trance allows you to make changes to your core beliefs and habits. Countless people have used hypnosis to quit smoking, get over trauma, focus, increase test-taking skills, eat healthier, and make more money, among other things – including addressing issues associated with your cancer. Hypnosis is probably one of the fastest ways to make changes to the subconscious mind.

But what happens when our subconscious has been affected in ways that are traumatic, or when we have a major emotional response to a person or event and don't fully process it and instead hold onto it in that great and unlimited repository of the subconscious? Understand that we have cancer cells in us; you have them in you. Your immune system deals with them, that is what the immune system does. Mutation happens, but something else happens to cause the cells to begin replicating out of control.

Dr. O. Carl Simonton had a theory. Dr. Simonton was an internationally acclaimed oncologist, author, and speaker who was best known for his pioneering insights and research in the field of psychosocial oncology. He earned his medical degree from the University of Oregon Medical School and then completed a three-year residency in radiation oncology, during which he developed a model of emotional support for the treatment of cancer patients, introducing the concept that one's state of mind could influence their ability to survive cancer.

Central to his method for engaging people's minds was his cancer development model. In the cancer development model, Dr. Simonton asserted that very strong emotions such as hopelessness, depression, and despair impair our coping mechanisms, and from both a conscious and unconscious perspective, we perceive death as a potential solution to our problems.

This mindset is recognized by the limbic system, which records these negative feelings of hopelessness. This information is then sent to the hypothalamus (remember Rossi's description of neurochemistry affecting cellular function in Chapter 2?), which translates it through neurotransmitters into messages that weaken and destabilize the immune system. This immune weakening has the effect of deregulating the pituitary gland. The endocrine system is thus compromised, and the result is an imbalance in adrenal hormones, which then makes the body susceptible to carcinogenic environmental influences.

That toxic emotions have the ability to destabilize our immune system makes sense, but now you have an explanation from a credible source. Feeling angry or enraged, sad, afraid, helpless, confused, depressed, terrified, inadequate, frustrated, ashamed, or embarrassed will weaken your immune system, expose you to the unmitigated toxicity of carcinogens that persist in your environment, and circumvent your body's defenses, which makes you susceptible to illness and disease.

Now you have a material explanation of Murphy's admonition to only give your subconscious positive suggestions. And you have an understanding of the subconscious' role in illness and disease. With this understanding as a baseline, Dr. Simonton's model of mind-body emotional support for cancer proposed reversing the model of cancer development using the same pathway, only in the opposite direction. Emotions and feelings are utilized to alter physiological conditions, erasing any feelings of hopelessness and strengthening the client's belief that they have a degree of control over their sickness and its eventual outcome (client, not patient, client is synonymous with the notion of active participant as we will cover in greater detail in Chapter 8, and is essentially the thesis of this book).

The theory goes that if the weakening of the immune system causes the illness, the contrary must logically be true. Is it a stretch to understand that a belief in recovery generates a feeling of hope and thereby strengthens your body's defenses? It is the very theory of expectancy that we discussed in the introduction. These feelings of hope are then recorded in the limbic system similar to the way the original stressors were recorded. The hypothalamus then receives the chemical expressions of hope, and, in turn, sends them to the pituitary gland, thus remobilizing your body's immune defenses. Hormonal balance restored, loop closed.

My healing journey really began when I first learned to meditate and go within, and then I gained a whole new understanding of the power of the mind by reading books by amazing teachers like Caroline Myss, Wayne Dyer, Deepak Chopra, Stephen Parkhill, Ernest Rossi, Kelly Turner, Joseph Murphy and so many others, many referenced throughout this book. I investigated the world of integrative medicine, including how hypnotherapy and the power of the subconscious mind can empower people with cancer to engage in their own healing and reverse the emotional underpinnings of disease. My instructor for hypnotherapy for cancer clients, Bruce Bonnett, who before becoming a hypnotherapist was a Harvard-trained attorney, gave me a book by Francisco Valenzuela, Ph. D., *Psycho-Oncology, Hypnosis and Psychosomatic Healing in Cancer*, in which Dr. Valenzuela detailed his use of hypnotherapy with cancer clients and introduced me to the Simonton model.

We briefly touched on hypnotherapy earlier in this chapter as a method for facilitating subconscious programming change. Hypnotherapy is an organic, non-invasive modality that in its deceptive simplicity unlocks the power of the subconscious mind. There is a growing body of research that establishes the efficacy of hypnotherapy in the cancer setting. I believe it is the missing thread in the fabric of care within the modern tumor model of care embraced by evidence-based medicine. I also believe that it is the wisdom of our ancient ancestors that you can benefit from tremendously, even in your modern, technologically influenced context.

Hypnotherapy, far from the stage and showmanship hypnosis that occupies so many people's perceptions, has grown as an integrative modality within the complementary or integrative care offerings of many hospitals. There is a growing body of research, much of it coming out of Stanford University, documenting the physiological explanations of what is at work within the brain in hypnosis, as well as the efficacy of its application as a complementary measure.

Unfortunately, as a society we tend to malign what we do not understand, and because hypnotherapy is deceptively simple, it is widely misunderstood. Consequently, hypnotherapy and, specifically hypnosis, tends to get a bad rap, and is a frequent easy target of Hollywood. Case in point is the recent movie *Get Out*, wherein it is used as a tool of manipulation and subjugation. Never mind that no one can be made to do anything against their will, but it makes for high theater! As a result, people can be reluctant to add hypnotherapy to their therapeutic plan.

Nevertheless, research is ongoing and hypnotherapy continues to be applied in beneficial ways. A report by the National Institutes of Health (NIH), for example, cites evidence supporting the efficacy of hypnosis for relief of chronic pain in cancer, irritable bowel syndrome, and tension headaches. In the cancer setting, hypnotherapy is used to reduce stress and anxiety, both conditions ever-present after a diagnosis, and typically throughout the recovery and healing process. The resolution of the stress and anxiety turn off the stress response and activate the relaxation response, which is where healing takes place. Beyond anxiety and stress reduction, hypnotherapy is also effective in facilitating therapeutic imagery journeys where the client visualizes healing. Also, hypnotherapy can be effective at releasing repressed emotions that many cancer clients tend to hold onto and that complicate healing.

In a study concluding in 2015 that included 150 participants, a researcher and nurse at the City of Hope Cancer Center found that 78 percent of those who used hypnosis experienced significant, lasting reduction in symptoms such as anxiety, pain, sleeplessness, fatigue, nausea, and vomiting.

In a journal article for clinicians entitled *Hypnosis for Cancer Care: Over 200 Years Young,* the authors noted that *Hypnosis has been used to provide psychological and physical comfort to individuals diagnosed with cancer for nearly 200 years.* The stated goals of the review were: 1) to describe hypnosis and its components and to dispel misconceptions; 2) to provide an overview of hypnosis as a cancer prevention and control technique – covering its use in weight management, smoking cessation, as an adjunct to diagnostic and treatment procedures, survivorship, and metastatic disease; and 3) to discuss future research directions. Overall, the literature supports the benefits of hypnosis for improving quality of life during the course of cancer and its treatment.

Dr. David Spiegel is Associate Chair of Psychiatry & Behavioral Sciences and Medical Director of the Center for Integrative Medicine at Stanford University School of Medicine, where he has been since 1975. Dr. Spiegel was also a lead investigator in an early study of Dr. Simonton's model, and recently has been at the forefront of research with the goal of exploring the simple question: what's going on in the brain when you're hypnotized? For some people, hypnosis is associated with loss of control or stage tricks, or the Hollywood representation noted above. But doctors like Spiegel know it to be a serious science, revealing the brain's ability to heal medical and psychiatric conditions.

Dr. Spiegel believes that hypnosis is the oldest Western form of psychotherapy, which is logical, as we know that Dr. Sigmund Freud used hypnosis before moving into psychoanalysis. He further believes that it's a very powerful means of changing the way we use our minds to control perception and our bodies, but he sometimes laments that *it's been tarred with the brush of dangling watches and purple capes.*

Hypnotherapy can be viewed as the ultimate therapeutic partnership, a relationship that forms between a client and a hypnotherapist that empowers the client to take ownership of their own healing. In this partnership, healing can be fully realized when clients become active participants in the development of their therapeutic plan. A repeated theme throughout this book – and in fact suggested by its very title – is that as an active participant in your healing and recovery through complete involvement in your therapeutic plan, you will feel more in control of your own health and are more likely to make sustained lifestyle changes that will lead you to improved health.

Hypnotherapy is a simple, yet powerful tool that has a long history of application in the cancer setting and definitely should be a part of your therapeutic plan. As we bring this chapter to a close however, there is one last note about the tools of your subconscious mind: *intuition*.

Survivors detailed in *Radical Remission* are reported to believe that the body has an innate, intuitive knowledge about what it needs in order to heal and often can let you know why you got sick in the first place. This is the fundamental reason that you must not yield control over your care to someone else and why your recovery depends on your active involvement. The homeostasis that characterizes the desire of the subconscious toward health and wellness can reveal important information if you are able to *trust your gut*, or listen to your intuition.

Intuition will come to you through a variety of ways, like a physical feeling. We have all had the experience of having a gut feeling. If something doesn't seem right, it probably isn't. Or information can come to you through meditation, dreams, or hypnosis, which you need to be paying attention to even though in the fog of stress, uncertainty, medication affects, and the million things going on in your life, it can seem trivial.

You want the powerful subconscious on *your* team and not working against you.

My intuition led me to understand that I needed to add spirituality to my life as I faced my cancer challenge. It also led me to understand the need for an Eastern influence to my journey and led me to a very influential yogi who gave me perspective and taught me so many useful and positive tools for self-care and self-realization. In the middle of my cancer treatment, my endocrinologist, one of the best in the Sacramento area and a very experienced and caring physician, was diagnosed with leukemia and I felt anguish for him even as I fought my own battle, but what followed was a series of other physicians who filled in for him trying to keep his practice operational and meet the needs of his many patients. The experience was disruptive and led to disconnected, disjointed care and advice, and my body paid the price as I was whip-sawed between hypo- and hyperthyroidism.

I knew I had to take charge of my overall care. I stepped up my meditation, and I had a session of hypnotherapy that helped me visualize my healing and recovery. I deepened my spirituality, as I have noted, and I radically changed my diet. I dove deep into my experiences and came to terms with repressed, painful emotions. I embraced a reason to live and moved past the fear-based notion of not wanting to die. Essentially, my intuition, hypnotherapy, and harnessing the power of my subconscious mind led me to all of the measures outlined in this book. The result? Cancer-free for six years. But the biggest challenge for me today as I spread the word about these powerful tools, share my story, and help people facing their own challenge is to get people to realize their power, to raise their hand and say, *yes, I'm ready to take charge.*

Are you ready?

CHAPTER 7
LET GO

"Unexpressed emotions will never die. They are buried alive and will come forth later in uglier ways."
Sigmund Freud

When a grain of sand or other foreign material gets inside an oyster, the oyster responds with an extraordinary process for addressing this constant irritation, a defense mechanism developed to protect the oyster from the foreign body. You may think pearls to be very beautiful, but the oyster usually loses its life to yield the pearl.

When you experience a traumatic event or a troubling emotion, your response is critical to your mental and physical well-being. This may sound obvious, but in reality, most people do not process their troubling emotions and instead suppress and repress them because they are difficult to deal with, create stress and anxiety, and distract you from your otherwise busy life. You go about your business not thinking consciously about this emotion that is tucked away, out of sight, but your subconscious knows it's there. These emotions can fester for years. This is the basis for the Simonton model of cancer development. These unresolved emotions create a chemical chain reaction that culminates in a compromised immune system.

It is human nature that we store up emotions and thoughts we are unable to deal with at the time until we are ready to let go of them, but it is not human nature for us to hold onto negative emotions because the homeostasis sought by the subconscious mind is to let experiences go. This is why an imbalance occurs and the immune system suffers. Psychologists have explained how these repressed emotions can be measured along neural pathways and how, by measuring electrical impulses along these pathways, repressed emotions show up as blockages along the pathways within the nervous system.

In his book *Answer Cancer*, Stephen Parkhill makes the case that there has been what he calls an initial sensitizing event, an emotional event or trauma that you did not process and that on top of which begin to stack up subsequent sensitizing events, or subsequent unresolved emotions. These subsequent events manifest in symptoms of illness like bursitis, asthma, or cancer, or habits such as nail biting or self-destructive behavior. Parkhill tells us that this symptom collection is the realm of the medical doctor who becomes what he calls an illness manager. If you are in pain, they numb it; if infected, they prescribe antibiotics; if you have a tumor, they cut it out. What he suggests instead is to use hypnotherapy to regress the client back to the initial event. This is Parkhill's corollary to the Simonton model of reversing the tumor development by bolstering the immune system, with the key difference that regression to cause is a bit more detailed and direct than simply applying positive suggestions of transformation. In other words, digging out underlying emotional events through regression hypnotherapy instead of just adding positive new sentiments over the top of what are sometimes deep-seated emotions. In either case, what you get is a restored immune system through the processing of emotions.

If you take a symptomatic approach, you can find that a symptom is muted, only to have another symptom crop up, resulting in an unending game that eventually just gets labeled chronic illness.

Carolyn Myss produced a must-see video years ago that's still available on the Internet. It's called *Why People Don't Heal*. In the video, she says that when she first became a medical intuitive and started working with people, she believed that everyone wanted to heal. We will go into this in greater detail in Chapter 10, but what she found is that healing can be very irrational. Why is healing irrational? Because, as Myss articulates, in order to heal, you must forgive, but this is not intuitive; it's indirect, and frankly it is hard for some people. Like the Simonton model and Parkhill's regression to cause, Myss believes the pathway to healing is through the emotions, and that the key emotion is forgiveness.

What she found, she says, is that many people are addicted to their wounds. It can provide a way to interact with and even control people. If a wounded person is confronted about their lack of performance or accountability, all they have to do is pull out their wound and, suddenly, they get sympathy and a built-in excuse for not performing.

Myss says, *pay attention to how you invest your energy*. If you invest your energy into a negative past, it is like trying to keep a corpse alive because the past is *dead*. You are trying to make a dead past provide your body with life force energy, but what you will be doing is draining your life force by trying to keep your dead past alive. This is referred to as *secondary gain*, which is defined as the advantage that occurs secondary to stated or real illness. Transition into the sick role may have some incidental secondary gains for patients. Types of secondary gain include using illness for personal advantage, exaggerating symptoms, consciously using symptoms for gain, and unconsciously presenting symptoms with no physiological basis. These symptoms may contribute to social breakdown and the patient's choice to remain sick. Sometimes there is a reason someone holds on to a limiting belief or an illness because they derive some perceived benefit from it, and usually not consciously.

You might see this as two sides to the same coin: suppressed immune system by way of repressed emotions versus lack of healing from loss of energetic life force. In either case, the result is illness and disease, and the solution leads to a restored immune system, health, and recovery.

That repressed emotions are at the core of illness is not a new idea. Freud said that repressed emotion was the cornerstone on which psychoanalysis exists and had sought to get patients to *consciously* resurrect their repressed emotions that he believed were the basis for their neuroses and led to disease as well as antisocial and self-destructive behavior. This desire that Freud had to flush out the repressed emotion into the realm of the conscious was the point at which he departed from his early use of hypnosis and established his psychoanalytical school of thought. But with all due respect for the amazing foundational work of Sigmund Freud and his colleagues and his successors, repression is a defense mechanism meant to protect you from the pain of the avoided emotion, and very few can openly face and confront that pain in a conscious and lasting fashion. Is it impossible? No. And imagine the satisfaction of the psychoanalyst who is able to get someone to come out from hiding, face and contend with their deepest, darkest repressed emotion! The reality is that most people would prefer to remain in hiding and swallow a chemical band-aid, rationalizing that drug therapy is correcting a chemical imbalance.

There was a story of a woman who presented to many different doctors with vague symptoms of on-again, off-again weakness and numbness that appeared first in one area, then in another. She had been told that it was all in her head, leaving her feeling dejected over the notion that what she was feeling was a figment of her imagination, despite it being very real to her. When another doctor did a complete workup and told her that she had an incurable disease that would eventually result in death, she felt relieved that it wasn't all in her head. Rather than be judged as a hypochondriac, having doctors give up on her and feeling helpless, she preferred a fatal diagnosis.

Understanding the impact of unresolved negative emotions is critical to your healing and recovery no matter what approach you take, and the investigation into the various approaches will not only inform you as to what is right for you, but may even trigger an intuitive, gut feeling that you should pay attention to.

Conversely, fostering positive emotions can be tonic for the soul and the subconscious. Take laughter, for example. Studies show that laughter activates the immune system. In one study, the physiological response produced by belly laughter was opposite of what is seen in classical stress, supporting the conclusion that cheery laughter is a eustress state – a state that produces healthy or positive emotions.

Research results further indicate that, after exposure to humor, there is a general increase in activity within the immune system, including: an increase in the number and activity level of natural killer cells that attack viral-infected cells and some types of cancer and tumor cells; an increase in activated T cells (T lymphocytes); an increase in the antibody IgA (immunoglobulin A), which fights upper respiratory tract infections; an increase in gamma interferon, which tells various components of the immune system to *turn on*; an increase in IgB, the immunoglobulin produced in the greatest quantity in your body, as well as an increase in Complement 3, which helps antibodies to pierce dysfunctional or infected cells – the increase in IgB and Complement 3 was not only present while subjects watched a humor video, there was also a lingering effect that continued to show increased levels the next day.

Take, for example, the case of Norman Cousins, an American political journalist, author, and professor who, in 1964, was given a few months to live. He had Ankylosing Spondylitis, a rare disease of the connective tissues. He was told that he had a 1 in 500 chance of survival and to *get his affairs in order*. But Cousins would have none of it, and among the steps he made to take charge of his healing plan, he got a number of funny movies including the Marx Brothers and *Candid Camera* shows. He invested a great deal of time watching these films and *laughing*, but he didn't just laugh. Although painful, he made a point of laughing until his stomach hurt.

Did it work? Who knows. Cousins finally died on November 30, 1990, 26 years after his doctors first delivered the seemingly devastating diagnosis. Can it be proved that laughing added 26 years to Norman Cousins' life? Probably not, but it's not a stretch to believe that because it strengthens the immune system that fights disease, laughter was a powerful tool that he utilized as part of his therapeutic plan.

Laughter, love, joy, happiness, and forgiveness. These are the emotions that you want to concentrate on, develop, nurture, and expand. Can it be difficult when faced with the cancer state and all of the myriad stresses, doubts, worries, and fears that accompany this diagnosis? Sure. But if there is a conscious decision to take as many effective actions as you can within your personal plan for healing and recovery, few are as positive, within reach, and naturally beneficial as the medicine within your own cabinet of emotions.

I had a client named Bob who was a union camera operator for 30 years in television and movies. He had a rare blood cancer and was struggling with the many medications he had to take and how they made him feel. Like most cancer clients, he also faced some fear.

When he first came in, we spent a great deal of time going over his history and experiences. He had had a great life up to this point, and after much thought, could not come up with a painful, deep emotional or traumatic experience from his life. I found it hard to believe, but didn't tell him that.

I decided to approach it differently. I asked if he had ever had a bitter disappointment. He thought for a moment, and then the light went on. He then proceeded to share with me that despite an illustrious career replete with union leadership roles, he had been on a set and the producer was very hands-on and took over his camera. It had been a long day, and they were shooting into the night. With nothing to do because his camera had been taken over, he fell asleep. When he was found to be sleeping, it didn't matter that someone else was working the camera, he was fired. He felt deeply ashamed and embarrassed. So ashamed and embarrassed that he took an early retirement, and despite still loving what he did all of his entire adult life as a career, left for the pasture.

Working through this disappointment allowed Bob to release these repressed emotions, and his health improved.

Don't be afraid to dive deep, dig some of this stuff up, and let it go. We all have these experiences, and we all repress them to some degree. It is your willingness to explore and release them that will free you from these ticking time bombs of the subconscious that are making you sick. Their release will set you free.

Exercise

In order to consciously explore what you might be holding on to, ask yourself the following questions and make a written record of your answers. Take your time, as this may be difficult. Reflect afterwards and revise as necessary. The goal is to learn from your experience and possibly identify what you may be holding onto so that you can begin the process of understanding, forgiving, and letting go. Then ask yourself what emotions you can direct positive emphasis to in order to light up your immune system.

Personal Inventory of High Stress Events

✓ What were the high stress events in your life that occurred in the year or two prior to your diagnosis or recurrence?

✓ What were your major emotional responses to these events?

✓ How could you have changed these conditions?

✓ How could you have changed your emotional response?

Personal Inventory of Positive Emotions Within Your Reach

✓ What can increase your happiness?

✓ What will bring you laughter, love?

✓ What can you do to bring yourself joy? What can you do to bring joy to others?

✓ What does happiness mean to you?

✓ Make a list of those you need to forgive, include yourself. Then make a decision to embrace forgiveness and really mean it.

CHAPTER 8
O CAPTAIN! MY CAPTAIN!

"When you take charge of your life, there is no longer need to ask permission of other people or society at large. When you ask permission, you give someone veto power over your life."
Albert F. Geoffrey

Until you hear the words, *you have cancer*, you can never fully understand the series of events, the physical and mental impacts, and the complete influence on your life the words can have. Your life is forever changed. In that moment, you have a choice. You can delay making the choice, but that, too, is a choice. Wayne Dyer used to speak of the *gap*, that moment between action and reaction. He believed that this is where your power lies, because in that moment you can choose your course of action. This is very similar to Viktor Frankl's suggestion that between stimulus and response, there is a space. In that space is your power to choose your response. In your response lies your growth and your freedom.

In your case, when you hear those words, you can choose to turn yourself over to a highly educated, extensively trained individual who is quite capable of understanding the physiological nature of your condition and the high percentage therapies that are recommended to give you the greatest possible chance of survival, which is compelling, or you can decide in that moment that no one has your well-being and best interests at heart more than you do and your best chances of a desirable outcome rest with your control over your care.

For me the gap was wide, like several months between hearing the words *you have cancer* and experiencing the disjointed care that followed my endocrinologist's leukemia diagnosis and led me to conclude that I had to be the one in charge.

Taking charge is not to say do not see your doctors or put a great deal of faith in their training and their ability. In fact, believing in your medical team and holding the expectation that you have capable medical practitioners on your side is critical to positive outcomes. What it does mean is that because you are the one with so much at stake, no one but you can appreciate the gravity of the situation. It means that after your office or hospital visit, when you go home and don't have access to the wealth of your doctors' training and education, you have to navigate your course. Build a file, do research, consider second opinions, understand what alternatives exist, and become well-informed about every aspect of your cancer. It is in this way that you can fully evaluate what you are being told.

Physicians need not be threatened by the body's ability to heal itself, or your conscious decision to be in charge of your therapeutic plan. There is data that suggests that patients need doctors or healers, but they need them to be a healing force, not a force of fear or pessimism. You need your doctors to offer positive belief and nurturing care, rather than threatening you with negative news, which merely enables the nocebo effect that we covered in Chapter 2.

The word *patient* is from Latin patientia – enduring, *suffering, submission*. Just as the Western medicine description of meditation in Chapter 2 is completely incongruent with the purpose of meditation, being labeled as suffering and a submissive is completely the wrong mindset for the task you have before you. Again, you need to be that person who does independent research, the person who asks questions and does not settle for spoon-feeding of information and condescension during brief, inadequate office visits. This will be the most important task of your life, and your life will literally depend on it. You are the person who must work to get well again. You are the central character, and you need to put yourself in charge.

Making yourself the team captain doesn't mean you are going it alone, it means that you are the leader of the team. The team includes physicians, surgeons, nurses, technicians, and family members. You can't do it without them, but they cannot *do it for you*. This is an important point, because if you turn yourself and your healing and recovery over to someone else, you will be missing the key ingredient in the process, and that is you. All of the preceding actions to reactivate your immune system will seem inauthentic to your powerful subconscious if you are unwilling to take the driver's seat.

A team is a good analogy because there will be many people involved in your experience from your primary care physician to specialists in radiation, pathology, oncology, and surgeons, as well as many mental health providers, social workers, nurses, technicians, and administrators. Believe it or not, they don't always talk to each other, and when they do, it isn't always the most efficient communication. These are busy people, and the teams come together in often ad hoc ways, not necessarily coordinated. The common thread that unites them all is *you,* and this is yet another important reason why you must be the captain.

I was forced to take charge because my doctor got sick and his fill-ins fumbled. Before this, while I investigated the surgeon and the endocrinologist who were recommended, I asked the referring physicians about who they were referring me to and why. I took notes. Sometimes, I was bothersome and irritated these busy people with my questions and my desire for complete explanations, but I didn't care, it was my skin in the game. When I could no longer rely on the main care providers, I researched all endocrinologists in the area, knew who was in plan and out of plan, and eventually got a waiver to see a physician who I trusted even though she was not in network. I also discovered that generally, women physicians tend to take more time, be more communicative, and have just a bit more compassion. I asked nuclear medicine doctors many questions, asked ultrasound techs what size the tumor was even though I knew their answer was going to be that they couldn't tell me, I would need to ask the doctor; I asked anyway and I got them to tell me. I didn't let scan techs bully me. I conferenced my primary care physician in with other providers because I trusted him and his knowledge. He had figured out what was wrong with me very early in the game and counseled me through the process, and I was fortunate enough that he would help me decipher what others told me.

It wasn't easy. And it won't always be easy for you; you are going to meet resistance. A certain paternalism pervades the medical community because of their education and knowledge and because they have seen a lot of people and how they act when they are sick. They have seen people who hold onto their illness as part of their identity, using it for primary and secondary gain, as noted in Chapter 7. It is difficult to deal with sickness day in and day out and not become a little jaded. This doesn't mean that they don't care; it just means that you always have to be in charge.

There is another factor that seldom gets talked about, but is a critical component to the nature of health care. If you hire a lawyer or an accountant, they work for you and you pay them. If they do not do a good job, you fire them and hire another. This is accountability. But in health care, it is different. There is usually someone else who pays for it, like your employer, although with the recent passage of the Affordable Care Act, we see for the first time a mandate on the individual to carry insurance. Nevertheless, you don't negotiate with a doctor for care. There are provider networks, and these provider networks contract with administrators in health maintenance organizations or preferred provider organizations, or in some cases old-fashioned insurance companies. The point is that healthcare is diffused; you don't pay for it directly and you don't negotiate for it, so you end up with an evidence of coverage that you don't understand and a system devoid of accountability as that term is understood in any other walk of life or economic sector. Have you ever looked at a hospital bill? The hospital charges 15 times the actual cost, the HMO pays one-ninth of the charges, disallows two-sevenths of the remainder, assigns the patient one-fifth in the form of a copay and another one-fifth if the patient hasn't met their deductible.

This system is frustrating and difficult almost by design. This is all the more reason to be in charge of your care and steadfast about requiring some form of accountability. But accountability is a two-way street, and just as you need to stay on top of your healthcare team, you need to hold yourself accountable, too.

Better health is an outcome of a better self. Caring for your body and taking charge of your health can be preventive as well as restorative. While healthcare providers and others can provide the needed guidance about health, disease, and treatment, it is ultimately you that matters. Accepting the guidance provided and implementing the steps is your responsibility.

Learning to meditate will be difficult at times and will require both time and effort on your part. Making significant and lasting changes to your diet will not be easy either; your eating habits have likely developed over a lifetime, and you are going to need to be more conscious about what you eat and drink than at any other time in your life. Deepening your spirituality won't be as difficult *per se*, but it will require a commitment to consistency in order to be effective. Working with your subconscious and your emotions are going to bring up difficult emotions at times and you will need to be strong and committed and, frankly, honest with yourself. And there will be times when you don't want to be the captain of the team, you will wonder if you can't just turn it all over to someone else who can just tell you what to do and where to go; and having a reason to live will require effort.

Being the team captain will not be easy, but it will be worth it. You are worth it and deserve nothing less than *your* very best. There is something about leadership that gets peoples' attention. Natural leadership doesn't push people; it inspires people to follow and is demonstrated by example. What you want to avoid, however, is being pushy or bossy. You want to communicate lovingly and listen openly. This is how team captains prepare themselves for leading the team. When you take charge of your healthcare, it demonstrates to people that you are serious about healing and recovery, including you.

What you will find is that as you push past the early difficult stages of making these changes, with time, it will get easier. Your commitment to yourself, with practice and patience, will become habit, and once habits are developed, before you know it, you have made a new way of life. And as you develop a new way of life, you will look at the research differently. You will look at the statistics differently. You will look at yourself differently. And your healthcare team will know you are committed to your own healing.

You should consider starting a journal. Think of it as a *captain's log*. There is increasing research pointing to the fact that regular journaling strengthens immune cells. Other research indicates that journaling decreases the symptoms of certain illnesses. Researchers have theorized that writing about stressful events helps you come to terms with them, thus reducing the impact of these stressors on your physical health.

Scientific evidence supports that journaling provides other unexpected benefits. The act of writing accesses your left brain, which is analytical and rational. While your left brain is occupied, your right brain is free to access that critical intuition that you should be tuning in to. At the very least, journaling helps you better understand yourself, others, and the world around you, including your healthcare journey. Some of the benefits of journaling include clarifying your thoughts and feelings; getting to know yourself better; reducing stress, and problem solving.

That this book has been titled *Take Charge of Your Cancer* should give you an appreciation for the importance of this step. With that said, however, this is a decision that is important, based upon the attitude and positioning developed sequentially, and the true benefits of being in charge will be realized after you have mastered the preceding five steps.

CHAPTER 9
REASON FOR LIVING

*"Everything can be taken from a man but
one thing: the last of human freedoms – to choose
one's attitude in any given set of circumstances,
to choose one's own way."*
Viktor Frankl

Viktor Frankl, M.D. Ph. D., was a Professor of Neurology and Psychiatry at the University of Vienna whose life was shaped by his experience in German concentration camps of the Second World War. After, he wrote *Man's Search for Meaning* and developed a form of existential analysis that he called *Logotherapy* based upon his firsthand observation that the people who had hope and found purpose and meaning were more likely to survive the camps than those who had no purpose for living because they had lost all hope and found no meaning in life.

Frankl believed that man's search for meaning was the primary motivation of his or her life. He dismissed the notion that a desire for meaning was a secondary rationalization of instinctual drives. There is no *universal* meaning, rather meaning is individual, and each person's meaning is unique and can only be fulfilled by themselves. Only this self-fulfillment can satisfy a person's desire for, and will to, meaning. He rebuffed those who would relegate a desire for meaning to defense mechanisms, reaction formations, and sublimations, and asked, *would you die for a defense mechanism?*

That someone was willing to die for something that they believed in, which ultimately gave meaning to their life, gave substance to the quest for meaning for Frankl and made its pursuit tangible. Yet, while being willing to die for your values and ideals makes the drive toward meaning real and substantive, its true value is when it is applied to the will to live.

It is not enough to not want to die, though. This is a fear-based motivation with death as the object, even if it is the object to be avoided. When death holds the central place in the goal, negative emotions are created and stimulated. Instead, all of the steps that we have covered to this point in this book are all reinforced, all turbocharged and all put into action by the overarching sentiment of having a reason to live. Remember the important role of expectation.

This may all sound grand in theory, but it can be difficult in practice as you face the challenge of cancer. What you will find, however, is that when you learn to meditate and go within, when you deepen your spirituality, when you release long-held yet unresolved emotions, you begin to see yourself and your life differently. Meaning will become apparent. But it will be a deeper meaning than the initial grasping desperation of trying to assign meaning to the fact that you got cancer.

When I discovered my then-wife's infidelity on top of my cancer, I considered, for a moment, taking my own life, or just succumbing to the cancer, thinking for a nano-second that it was all just too much to bear. Then I thought of my children, reason enough to want to live and see them blossom – I now have a grandchild. And then a new vision of myself emerged, and I knew I had unfinished business. This book is central to that unfinished business, as is building a practice to share what I have learned through hypnotherapy and coaching. In that moment, that gap, I realized that cancer wasn't my death sentence; it was my wake-up call, the vehicle for me to find meaning and purpose in my life. I want to help lead you to your own moment.

This is really all about you, and that is okay. Many people, like myself, derive their reason for living from family – children, grandchildren, spouses, and that is great. Or they have unfinished business. The most powerful motivator emerges when that unfinished business is you.

A diagnosis should encourage you to ask questions like *why is this happening to me?* Why right now? Not in the sense of feeling like a victim, but asking the question with a sense of openness and curiosity. Some people talk about and view their cancer as a wake-up call for them to take a close look at where they are in life; I know I did. It is so easy to let life become a treadmill that grinds you down. Were you feeling fulfilled or trapped? When life gets discouraging, it could be a huge opportunity to find and value your true self, your unheeded aspirations, and even your own basic needs.

You may have never thought it was possible or necessary to make any changes in your life prior to your diagnosis. Viewed differently through the lens of involuntary transformation, you can let cancer be a journey to lead you down a new and more fulfilling path in life. Let the journey lead you to your life purpose, even if you have no clue what that might be. You just might find the difference that you are meant to make in the world, which just might help you finally feel passionate and fulfilled, or more so than you thought you had been. Ask me how I know. This book is the beginning of a whole new journey for me, a journey filled with purpose and meaning. I now know why I got cancer.

CHAPTER 10
CONCLUSION

"To know yourself as the Being underneath the thinker, the stillness underneath the mental noise, the love and joy underneath the pain, is freedom, salvation, enlightenment."
Eckhart Tolle

Cancer is without a doubt one of the most challenging things you will face in your life. The experience brings with it the opportunity to stop, reflect, and make changes. If you are able to see the opportunity, you can make significant, life-enhancing changes that you may never have even considered before your diagnosis.

You will have many choices to make and much research to do. There are many resources out there and many cover some of the same ground. Sometimes the early experience of the subconscious work with intuition points you in the direction that is right for you. Listen to your intuition.

Every person with cancer has a unique journey, but all who follow this seven-step process share a desire to learn from those who applied these techniques to move through the different phases of transformation in order to activate their natural healing processes. If you can open up to and receive the inner guidance that comes through difficult situations, it could allow you to embrace the new opportunities that present themselves.

Worthy of note is the fact that these same techniques for taking charge of your cancer can work to prevent cancer and other disease. Imagine making a few lifestyle changes and heading disease off at the pass. In a day and age where fear drives decisions like a prophylactic mastectomy based upon a genetic predisposition, wouldn't it be a sign of self-respect to instead adopt self-care techniques that the only side effect of was to know and love yourself more and better and defend yourself against the onset of disease?

Those who take charge of their cancer will:

- ✓ Learn different tools and techniques using a mind, body, spirit approach
- ✓ Trust the amazing power of the subconscious
- ✓ Look at food in a whole new way
- ✓ Commit to lifestyle changes that demonstrate self-care
- ✓ Work through strong emotions
- ✓ Develop faith and deeper spirituality
- ✓ Understand and believe in the incredible healing power of your body
- ✓ Be curious and open

✓ Live in the present moment

✓ Learn to open up to your intuition

It is hard to leave you here because there are always so many more questions. My hope for you is that you use this guide to open your mind and your heart to seeing a different way to respond to your challenge and move away from fear and uncertainty. Know that this book, and my hypnotherapy and coaching practice, are all the result of adopting these techniques, embracing transformation, and finding my purpose by putting myself into the service of others. My further hope for you is that you, too, can embrace transformation by taking charge of your cancer.

ACKNOWLEDGEMENTS

We all dream of someday writing a book, but fulfilling the dream is very difficult as a practical matter, as everyone who has yet to complete theirs can attest. To get across the finish line, we need those who stand behind us, in front of us, and beside us.

My dream became a reality because Britt believed, Beth pushed, and Diane supported. And then there was Angela! Who knew I had so many books in me and that the reason I hadn't completed one was because I was trying to write them all at the same time. It is one thing to understand the principle of Occam's Razor and another thing altogether to put it into practice. Thank you all for helping my dream come true.

To the Morgan James Publishing team: Special thanks to David Hancock, CEO & Founder for believing in me and my message. To my Author Relations Manager, Gayle West, thanks for making the process seamless and easy. Many more thanks to everyone else, but especially Jim Howard, Bethany Marshall, and Nickcole Watkins.

I did not hear life's whisper, and so it yelled, and in that yell was the seed of my transformation, which turned out to be an unwrapped gift.

To the authors of the many books I read to come to an understanding of the power of our own involvement in healing and the mind-body connection, a heartfelt thank you for your groundbreaking work; your belief in the human mind, body, and spirit; and your willingness to share even when it wasn't always popular to do so.

And to all those who seek answers and wellness, my hope is that you find usefulness and inspiration from these pages. I hold encouragement and love for you.

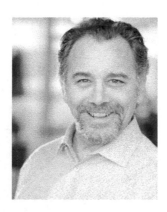

ABOUT THE AUTHOR

Norman Plotkin is a former lobbyist and cancer survivor who has found his passion for helping people through coaching, practicing hypnotherapy, speaking, and writing around wellness, healing, and recovery.

During a 25-year career in and around state government, Norman gained powerful insights into health policy and the internal workings of the practice of medicine as a committee consultant to the California State Assembly Health Committee and a lobbyist for the California Medical Association.

Norman is certified in hypnotherapy for cancer clients and has expanded his offering to include coaching on the seven proven factors that make a real difference for cancer patients, or anyone with chronic illness, for true healing and recovery. On his journey, he discovered that the power of the therapeutic partnership is established when people become active participants in the development of their therapeutic plan, because they feel more in control of their own well-being and are more likely to make sustained lifestyle changes to improve their health.

Norman's ultimate goal is that his experience and research will enable him to positively impact the lives of survivors and their families.

Norman has three children and a grandchild. One of his most amazing life experiences was taking his daughter through hypnobirthing, which resulted in a 24-minute delivery, delivering on his daughter's desire for natural childbirth without drugs! He lives in Oceanside, CA, where he can be found, when not seeing clients, cutting through traffic on his Yamaha.

Connect with Norman at:

www.NormanPlotkin.com

THANK YOU

Thanks so much for reading. The fact that you've gotten to this point in the book tells me something important about you: you're ready. You're ready to shift out of overwhelm and quit feeling like a helpless victim. You're ready to experience participation in and ownership of your cancer.

Please visit my website to inquire about helpful free checklists to keep you on track as you complete the *Take Charge* process: www.normanplotkin.com.

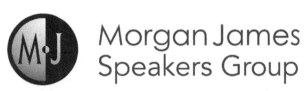

Morgan James
Speakers Group

➚ www.TheMorganJamesSpeakersGroup.com

We connect Morgan James published
authors with live and online events
and audiences who will benefit
from their expertise.

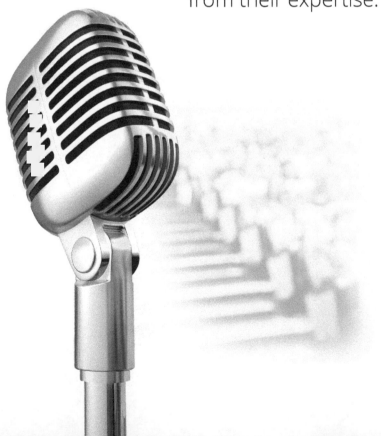

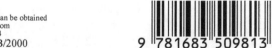